"Health workers were among the first and most impacted by COVID-19—not just by the virus, but also by the changes to rosters, leave, school attendance, and family impact. The authors conducted a wide-ranging survey that tapped into the concerns, challenges, and demands placed on our health workers, and their responses. This book provides a unique insight into the impact of the pandemic on a vital cohort; it illustrates some of the issues faced in the health system that have been exposed as a result of the pandemic, and the courage and resilience shown by many".

Ruth Vine, *Deputy Chief Medical Officer for Mental Health, Australia*

"While the whole society has been through a highly threatening and morale-sapping experience through the pandemic, healthcare workers have been at the eye of the storm. This book confirms that they have performed incredibly, suffered greatly, and also that the experience has changed so many in fundamental ways. This book provides a window into this experience, which is captured through the dedication and commitment of those who fought to conduct this unique survey. The healing professions offer the greatest vocation that can be followed and are deeply respected. This book shows why and reveals the deeply human elements of health and medical care under extreme conditions".

Patrick McGorry, AO, *Executive Director of Orygen and Professor of Youth Mental Health, University of Melbourne, Australia*

"Based on a rich and expansive data set, this book gives a fascinating insight into the experiences of health workers in the pandemic context. It reveals new challenges that emerged and illuminates existing cracks in the health system. This book provides an important opportunity to hear from healthcare workers in their words. Those who work in this sector will find solace in this book as a way of making sense of their experiences and giving voice to their emotions. For those in health policy or management roles, it is incumbent upon us to hear these voices and think about how we can shape the sector so that we learn from this experience".

Helen Dickinson, *Professor of Public Service Research, University of New South Wales, Australia*

"In his 1947 novel *The Plague*, Albert Camus wrote of 'All who, while unable to be saints but refusing to bow down to pestilences, strive their utmost to be healers'. *Experiences of Health Workers in the COVID-19 Pandemic* is a remarkable record of the experiences of Australian health workers. In the midst of fear, uncertainty, and exhaustion, their voices are an eloquent call for understanding, support, and recognition of our shared humanity in the face of a modern plague".

Ron Paterson, *Emeritus Professor of Health Law and Policy, University of Auckland, New Zealand*

EXPERIENCES OF HEALTH WORKERS IN THE COVID-19 PANDEMIC

Experiences of Health Workers in the COVID-19 Pandemic shares the stories of frontline health workers—told in their own words—during the second wave of the COVID-19 pandemic in Australia. The book records the complex emotions healthcare workers experienced as the pandemic unfolded, and the challenges they faced in caring for themselves, their families, and their patients. The book shares their insights on what we can learn from the pandemic to strengthen our health system and prepare for future crises.

The book draws on over 9,000 responses to a survey examining the psychological, occupational, and social impacts of COVID-19 on frontline health workers. Survey participants came from all areas of the health sector, from intensive care doctors to hospital cleaners to aged care nurses, and from large metropolitan hospitals to rural primary care practices. The authors organise these free-text responses thematically, creating a shared narrative of health workers' experiences. Each chapter is prefaced by a brief commentary that provides context and introduces the themes that emerged from the survey.

This book offers a unique historical record of the experiences of thousands of healthcare workers at the height of the second wave of the pandemic and will be of great interest to anyone interested in the experiences of healthcare workers, and the psychological, organisational, healthcare policy, and social challenges of the COVID-19 pandemic.

Marie Bismark is a professor of Law and Public Health in the Melbourne School of Population and Global Health at the University of Melbourne, Australia. She is also a public health physician, health law academic, and advanced trainee in psychiatry. During the pandemic, she provided mental health care to patients in the emergency department, intensive care unit, and COVID-19 wards of The Royal

Melbourne Hospital. She also leads a research team at the University of Melbourne, focused on the interface between patient safety and clinician wellbeing.

Karen Willis is professor of Public Health at Victoria University, Australia. She is a health sociologist and qualitative methodologist. She co-led the Australian Frontline Health Worker Survey and is currently co-leading the Future-Proofing the Frontline project to develop interventions to support health workers during times of crisis. Her previous research has examined how patients and professionals navigate the healthcare system, self-management of chronic conditions, and the experience of loneliness for people with chronic conditions. She is co-editor of *The Covid-19 Crisis: Social Perspectives* (Routledge, 2021) and co-editor of *Navigating Private and Public Healthcare: Experiences of Patients, Doctors and Policy-Makers* (Palgrave Macmillan, 2020).

Sophie Lewis is senior lecturer in the School of Health Sciences at the University of Sydney, Australia. She has an inter-disciplinary background in sociology and public health and her research uses innovative qualitative methods to explore the experience of living with long-term conditions. Her current research examines how people with chronic illnesses experience loneliness, self-management support in patient/clinician interactions, end of life care decision-making, and the experiences of living with advanced cancer.

Natasha Smallwood is associate professor in the Central Clinical School at Monash University, Australia, clinical associate professor at the University of Melbourne, Australia, and consultant respiratory physician at Alfred Health. Her research interests include symptom management, supporting patients with severe lung diseases, gender equity, and clinician wellbeing. She co-led the Australian Frontline Health Worker Survey and is currently co-leading the Future-Proofing the Frontline project to develop interventions to support health workers during times of crisis.

The COVID-19 Pandemic Series

This series examines the impact of the COVID-19 pandemic on individuals, communities, countries, and the larger global society from a social scientific perspective. It represents a timely and critical advance in knowledge related to what many believe to be the greatest threat to global ways of being in more than a century. It is imperative that academics take their rightful place alongside medical professionals as the world attempts to figure out how to deal with the current global pandemic, and how society might move forward in the future. This series represents a response to that imperative.

Series Editor: J. Michael Ryan

Titles in this Series:

COVID 19
Two Volume Set
Edited by J. Michael Ryan

COVID 19
Volume I: Global Pandemic, Societal Responses, Ideological Solutions
Edited by J. Michael Ryan

COVID 19
Volume II: Social Consequences and Cultural Adaptations
Edited by J. Michael Ryan

COVID-19: Social Inequalities Human Possibilities
J. Michael Ryan and Serena Nanda

Experiences of Health Workers in the COVID-19 Pandemic
In Their Own Words
Marie Bismark, Karen Willis, Sophie Lewis and Natasha Smallwood

Creative Resilience and COVID-19
Figuring the Everyday in a Pandemic
Edited by Irene Gammel and Jason Wang

COVID-19 and Childhood Inequality
Edited by Nazneen Khan

EXPERIENCES OF HEALTH WORKERS IN THE COVID-19 PANDEMIC

In Their Own Words

Marie Bismark, Karen Willis, Sophie Lewis, and Natasha Smallwood

Routledge
Taylor & Francis Group
LONDON AND NEW YORK

Cover image: © Getty Images

First published 2022
by Routledge
2 Park Square, Milton Park, Abingdon, Oxon OX14 4RN

and by Routledge
605 Third Avenue, New York, NY 10158

Routledge is an imprint of the Taylor & Francis Group, an Informa business

British Library Cataloguing-in-Publication Data
A catalogue record for this book is available from the British Library

Library of Congress Cataloging-in-Publication Data
Names: Bismark, Marie, 1973– author. | Willis, Karen, 1960– author. |
Lewis, Sophie, 1984– author. | Smallwood, Natasha, 1976– author.
Title: Experiences of health workers in the COVID-19 pandemic: in their
own words / Marie Bismark, Karen Willis, Sophie Lewis and Natasha Smallwood.
Description: Milton Park, Abingdon, Oxon; New York, NY: Routledge, 2022. |
Series: The COVID-19 pandemic series |
Includes bibliographical references and index. |
Identifiers: LCCN 2021044001 (print) | LCCN 2021044002 (ebook) |
ISBN 9781032132709 (hardback) | ISBN 9781032132716 (paperback) |
ISBN 9781003228394 (ebook)
Subjects: LCSH: Medical personnel–Job stress. |
Medical personnel–Psychology. | COVID-19 (Disease)
Classification: LCC RA410.7.B55 2022 (print) | LCC RA410.7 (ebook) |
DDC 362.11068/3–dc23/eng/20211108
LC record available at https://lccn.loc.gov/2021044001
LC ebook record available at https://lccn.loc.gov/2021044002

ISBN: 9781032132709 (hbk)
ISBN: 9781032132716 (pbk)
ISBN: 9781003228394 (ebk)

DOI: 10.4324/9781003228394

Typeset in Bembo
by Newgen Publishing UK

For the health workers of the COVID-19 pandemic, and for those who cared for the carers.

CONTENTS

FOREWORD

The COVID-19 pandemic has challenged, and led to the revision of, previously understood models of emotional response to disasters and catastrophic events. The journey through the pandemic has evoked a broad range of emotions, that regardless of our profession—or from whatever walk of life we come—we would rather not be feeling.

Whether this book is read straight through or "dipped into" it reminds readers how much we are indebted to all who work in healthcare at this time.

In visiting the experiences of healthcare workers, we are challenged to consider the core of our own humanity and confronted with the fragility of human existence and our own identity.

Fellow healthcare workers can find words that resonate with and validate their own experiences. The general public, whether or not they have needed to access healthcare during the pandemic, are reminded that all healthcare workers are more than their job. They have many roles outside the workplace that, like the rest of the community, have been impacted directly and indirectly by COVID.

The genesis of this book was a research project and the healthcare workers who participated were courageously honest and frank in their contributions. Their courage extended beyond sharing a story. They kept going at times despite feeling physically and psychologically unsafe, exhausted, or experiencing the effects of direct and vicarious trauma.

While, as individuals, as a community, or as healthcare policymakers, we do not want to dwell unduly on or get stuck in traumatic experiences, we cannot afford to forget the enormous learnings that come from the pandemic. Even though in Australia we have one of the best healthcare systems in the world, COVID showed us some of its imperfections. It is even more important than ever to ensure we have a healthcare system that has the wellbeing of its workers as a priority.

Dr Kym Jenkins
Chair of the Council of Presidents of Medical Colleges
Past-President of the Royal Australian New Zealand College of Psychiatrists
Chair of the Migrant and Refugee Health Partnership

Throughout history the human voices in stories have given meaning to experiences. The stories recorded in this book illuminate the long shadow that the COVID-19 pandemic has cast on healthcare workers and their families.

I congratulate Prof. Marie Bismark, Prof. Karen Willis, Dr Sophie Lewis and A/Prof. Natasha Smallwood for this work. With nearly 10,000 respondents, their research provides a rare window into the challenges that healthcare workers have faced during the COVID-19 pandemic in Australia.

We have each experienced our own unique roller-coaster of experiences during this pandemic: the sacrifices made, the fears for our own health and the health of others, the dread of transmitting the virus to others, juggling work and home schooling, or supporting family members. For some, the pandemic has had some silver linings too: the slower pace of life, time to reconnect with the simpler things in life, the sense of community pulling together, and the incredible teamwork that can emerge from adversity.

We have seen the good and the bad of social media. It has allowed us to connect with others when we cannot be together physically, and to keep up to date with new information and evidence. But sadly, we have also seen social media being used to misinform or mislead.

More than ever, this pandemic has shown us the value of taking care of ourselves and being kind to others. When someone is separated from their family and friends, at their time of need, the role you play as a healthcare worker—in providing care and compassion—is so important, even if it has to be from behind the barrier of PPE.

Hearing the stories of healthcare workers—in their own words—provides us all with a deeper understanding of the impact of the pandemic. I applaud everyone who has provided care during the pandemic, including those who took the time to share their experiences through this survey. The work you do is so very important.

Professor Alison McMillan
Chief Nursing and Midwifery Officer
Australian Government Department of Health

SERIES FOREWORD

When the SARS-CoV-2 virus began to alter the face of the world in early 2020, I set about pulling together a two-volume set of edited volumes to help add a social-scientific voice to pandemic understandings. It became obvious from the beginning that perhaps the most important players in this newly emerging pandemic world were healthcare workers. That said, their voices were going largely unheard and, worse yet, far too often ignored.

Following the success of my own two edited pandemic volumes, I have since become the series editor for Routledge's *The COVID-19 Pandemic Series* and was delighted, nay honoured, to quickly receive a proposal from Marie, Karen, Sophie, and Natasha for the book you are now reading. Their proposal promised to do what society has not by giving priority to the voices of those individuals most directly engaged in keeping us alive. The finished volume you hold in your hands has more than delivered on that promise.

The authors of this volume are all highly respected and well-known professionals in their field. Their combined decades of research have already gifted us with volumes of insights and knowledge, and this collective work has done no less. Combining their own professional insights with research drawn from the impressive "Australian COVID-19 Frontline Healthcare Workers study", this volume adds the all-important voice of frontline healthcare workers to our collective understanding of pandemic impacts and consequences. More than just another addition to the pandemic literature, this volume is a monument to the perspectives of those who have worked so tirelessly, and sacrificed so much, to try to save us from one of the most deadly viruses to infect humanity in the last century.

I am truly honoured to have this work as a part of the series, and grateful to Marie, Karen, Sophie, and Natasha not only for their own wonderful contributions to helping us better understand our ongoing COVID-19 world, but for also giving voice to those who have, and still are, so selflessly committing themselves to help rescue us from the SARS-CoV-2 virus.

J. Michael Ryan
Series Editor, The COVID-19 Pandemic Series

ACKNOWLEDGEMENTS

This book would not exist without the contributions of a great many people.

We thank the other members of the Australian COVID-19 Frontline Health Workers study team: Assoc. Prof. Leila Karimi (La Trobe University), Prof. Anne Holland (Monash University), Prof. Shyamali Dharmage (University of Melbourne), Dr Claire Long (Western Health), Dr Cara Moore (Royal Melbourne Hospital), Dr Nicole Atkin (Peter MacCallum Cancer Centre), Assoc. Prof. Mark Putland (Royal Melbourne Hospital & University of Melbourne), Assoc. Prof. Douglas Johnson (Royal Melbourne Hospital & University of Melbourne), Dr Irani Thevarajan (Royal Melbourne Hospital & University of Melbourne), Dr Irene Ng (Royal Melbourne Hospital), Ms Debra Sandford (University of Adelaide), Dr Elizabeth Barson (Royal Melbourne Hospital), Assoc. Prof. Tony McGillion (La Trobe University), and Assoc. Prof. Jane Munro (Royal Children's Hospital & University of Melbourne).

Thank you to our research assistants, Anu Tayal, Lauren Vickery, and Paulina Ezer, for their diligence and commitment. Paulina, you will always be a part of us.

We wish to thank the funders of the Australian COVID-19 Frontline Health Worker study: The Royal Melbourne Hospital Foundation and the Lord Mayor's Charitable Foundation. Additional funds for collating survey quotes into this book were provided by a National Health and Medical Research Council Investigator Grant awarded to Marie Bismark.

Rebecca Brennan was our publisher at Routledge, and we thank her for believing that these stories needed to be told.

Individually, Marie thanks her three children: Zoe who was the first to know when the idea for this book was formed in managed isolation, Stella for always bringing out the best in others, and Finn for asking great questions. She also thanks her husband Matthew, her parents Louw and Margriet, her Royal Melbourne Hospital colleagues (especially Marilyn, Kristi, and Patricia), her book club (which is more like a life club), and her psychiatry study group for their enduring kindness and care.

Karen thanks her supportive friends, family, and colleagues, especially Stuart, her partner in life, love, and lockdowns! Writing is also made easier with the support and love of sons and their partners: Marius and Ellie, and Dominic and Melinda; and the joyous distractions of grandchildren—Leo, Ethan, and Evie.

Sophie thanks her partner, friends, family, and colleagues for their continuous support.

Natasha thanks her husband David and their three children Isabella, James, and Emma for their infinite love and unfailing support of her clinical work and research.

And finally, and most importantly, we acknowledge the healthcare workers who faced the pandemic with their full humanity. Thank you for taking the time to share your experiences and ideas with us. We hope this book gives you the collective voice you asked for.

TERMS AND ABBREVIATIONS

This list has been compiled to assist readers who may not be familiar with the many different terms that are used to describe those who work in healthcare or the many different areas in which care is provided.

Acute care: hospital-based active, short-term treatment for an illness or injury.

Administrative worker: a clerical or administrative worker, including ward clerks, booking clerks, receptionists, secretaries, and practice managers.

Allied health assistant: someone who works under the supervision of (usually) an allied health practitioner.

Allied health practitioner: a trained healthcare professional who is not a dentist, doctor or nurse. Wherever possible in this book, we have specified the allied health profession (e.g., dietician, occupational therapist, orthoptist, pharmacist, physiotherapist, radiographer, speech therapist, social worker, psychologist)

Age: only the age range provided by each survey participant is reported.

Community care: care provided outside a hospital setting, including in a person's home, community-based clinic, or general practitioner's (GP) clinic.

COVID-19: coronavirus disease 2019, an infectious disease caused by the SARS-CoV-2 virus.

Dental practitioner: includes dentists, dental hygienists, dental therapists, dental prosthetists, and oral health therapists.

Environmental services: includes activities such as housekeeping, cleaning, waste disposal, and laundry.

Facilities and maintenance: people who keep spaces, structures, and infrastructure in good condition in healthcare settings such as hospitals.

Furlough: a mandatory, temporary leave of absence after exposure to COVID-19 virus.

General medicine: treatment of diseases affecting the internal organs, including complex chronic conditions, whose primary treatment does not involve surgery (similar to internal medicine).

General practitioner: a specialist in general practice (similar to a primary care physician or family practice doctor).

Hot zone: area for assessment and treatment of people with suspected or confirmed COVID-19.

JobKeeper: financial support provided by the Australian government to businesses significantly impacted by the pandemic to enable them to continue paying their employers.

Junior doctor: a doctor who has not yet completed specialist training including interns, residents, and registrars (sometimes referred to as house officers, trainees, or advanced trainees).

Manager: a person responsible for leading and controlling a team of people, including departmental (also known as unit) and organisational directors.

Medical scientist: a person who performs medical tests on blood, other body fluids, or tissues, or assesses muscle or nerve function, to assist clinicians in the diagnosis, treatment, and prevention of disease.

Medical specialty: including but not limited to neurology, gastroenterology, endocrinology, haematology, rheumatology, renal medicine, oncology, cardiology, neurology, palliative care, and paediatrics. Some other medical specialties are specifically listed in participants' information (e.g., respiratory medicine or aged care).

N95 mask: a mask that filters at least 95% of airborne particles when properly fitted

Non-clinical: a healthcare worker whose role does not involve direct patient care.

Nursing casual pool: nurses who are allocated to work in different parts of the hospital with the greatest need (similar to bank nurses). These nurses may or may not work regularly in one particular hospital area.

Perioperative care: the care provided at any time around a patient's surgical procedure including ward admission, anaesthesia, surgery, and recovery.

Phlebotomist: a nurse or other healthcare worker trained in drawing blood for testing or donation.

PPE: personal protective equipment.

Residential aged care facility: a home for older people who can no longer live at home or need help with everyday tasks (similar to nursing home).

Respiratory medicine: the prevention, diagnosis, and treatment of disease affecting the respiratory (breathing) system.

Respiratory scientist: a clinical physiologist who performs tests to measure lung or sleep function, for example, in patients with asthma or chronic obstructive pulmonary disease. See also medical scientist.

SARS-CoV-2: severe acute respiratory syndrome coronavirus 2.

Senior doctor: a doctor who has completed several years of postgraduate specialist training and who holds specialist postgraduate qualifications in a specific area of medicine (e.g., a consultant, specialist, or senior staff specialist).

Stage Four Lockdown: the public health measures imposed during the second wave of the pandemic in the state of Victoria, Australia, which included stay at home orders for all but essential work, medical care, compassionate care, one hour of exercise within a five-kilometre radius, and obtaining groceries (one person per household per day), no indoor or outdoor gatherings of more than two people unless all are from the same household, remote learning for all school children (with some exceptions for children of essential workers), closure of all non-essential services and venues including gyms, restaurants, cinemas, and hairdressers, a curfew between 8pm and 5am, and closure of state and international borders with a requirement for 14 days of hotel quarantine.

Subacute aged care: a level of care between community/residential and hospital aged care.

Support staff: healthcare workers who support the day-to-day running of health facilities (usually hospitals). See also facilities administrative, environmental services and facilities management.

Surgical: includes general surgery, orthopaedics, cardiothoracic surgery, ear, nose and throat surgery, plastic surgery, urology, neurosurgery, paediatric surgery, vascular surgery, obstetrics, and gynaecology.

Technician: a person who carries out a range of tasks to assist professional clinical staff. Tasks may be patient-related, relate to technical equipment, or working in a medical laboratory.

WorkCover: government compensation for workplace acquired injuries (including infections).

1

INTRODUCTION

> I feel I'm living between two worlds. Those who work in healthcare and understand the stress of working in a COVID environment, and those who don't. I feel that if the general public knew what it was like to work in constant fear of passing on the virus to their loved ones, they would feel differently about restrictions on the way we live. I feel my family don't understand the pressure I'm under every day.
>
> *Nurse, surgical, female, age 41–50*

Healthcare workers enter their profession with a deep commitment to serving others. From emergency department nurses to medical specialists to disability support workers, there is a shared commitment to caring for people in times of need. Yet healthcare workers also experience high workplace demands and stressors in their day-to-day lives. The work can be unpredictable and unrelenting. Despite every effort to preserve life and health, some patients will never fully recover and some will die. Healthcare workers go to work each day, hoping to make a positive difference, in the face of financial constraints, staffing shortages, heavy expectations, and strong emotions.

Given all these issues, it is unsurprising that working in healthcare takes its toll. Doctors and nurses, in particular, are known to suffer from higher rates of burnout, anxiety, depression, and suicide than other occupations. The wellbeing of healthcare workers matters to individual workers and their families and, more broadly, affects the quality of care, patient safety, and workforce retention.

While healthcare workers in Australia are used to responding to crises such as bushfires, floods, mass casualty accidents, and outbreaks of disease, the current COVID-19 pandemic is a crisis of a scale not seen since the Spanish Influenza that followed World War I. In countries around the world, COVID-19 has interrupted daily life, made normal work practices and routines impossible, and given rise to

DOI: 10.4324/9781003228394-1

fear and uncertainty. Indeed, our very language has changed to include new phrases such as "social distancing" and "COVID-normal". Unsurprisingly, the pandemic has had a profound effect on the physical, emotional, economic, and social well-being of populations globally.

For healthcare workers, this situation has been no different, except that work cannot suddenly stop and there have been multiple new challenges. Around the world, people providing patient care in hospitals and the community have had to respond quickly to heavy workloads, large volumes of new information, new work practices and roles, redeployment or job insecurity, separation from loved ones, and increased risks to their own lives and the lives of family members.

The Australian COVID-19 Frontline Healthcare Workers study

After earlier pandemics, such the 2003 outbreak of severe acute respiratory syndrome (SARS), research showed that the mental health of many healthcare workers suffered, with potentially long-lasting effects. Similarly, a growing body of evidence—from around the world—is finding high rates of anxiety, depression, post-traumatic stress, and burnout among healthcare workers during the COVID-19 pandemic. Importantly, some healthcare workers are more vulnerable to these harms, and both personal and workplace factors can contribute to this risk.

With this knowledge, our research team believed it was vital to understand the psychosocial, workplace, and financial effects of the COVID-19 pandemic on healthcare workers in Australia. We hoped that this knowledge would help with recognising their needs, developing practical solutions, and supporting the health workforce during crises now and in the future. And so, the "Australian COVID-19 Frontline Healthcare Workers study" was born.

The survey was a voluntary, anonymous, online survey of healthcare workers in hospitals, general practice, and community care across Australia. We invited workers from all health roles (doctors, nurses, allied health, medical laboratory, administrative, and other support staff) to take part. The survey was shared by leaders at hospitals and community organisations, professional colleges, societies and associations, universities, government health departments, newspapers, television, radio, and social media.

The survey ran from August to October 2020, which coincided with the second wave of the pandemic in Australia. Throughout this time, international arrivals into Australia and interstate travel were largely halted. Severe lockdown restrictions were in place in the state of Victoria including: mandatory mask-wearing, travel limited to five kilometres from home, an evening curfew, a one-hour daily limit for outdoor exercise, working from home for all but essential workers, home-schooling, restrictions on seeing extended family, the closure of most shops, hospitality and entertainment venues, and shutting of interstate and international borders. During the second wave, around 20,000 people in Australia were infected with COVID-19 and around 800 died. These numbers were many times lower than similar countries overseas. Nevertheless, healthcare workers were disproportionately affected, with thousands of healthcare workers becoming infected with COVID-19 at work. It would be another four months before the first vaccine against COVID-19 was provisionally approved for use in Australia.

It was in this context that healthcare workers were invited to contribute to our survey. Healthcare workers generally are reluctant to participate in surveys for many reasons, including lack of time. However, within eight weeks we had received almost 10,000 responses from healthcare workers across Australia, which was a truly incredible response. We heard from people working in all roles and areas of the health sector, ranging from aged care nurses to hospital cleaners to intensive care specialists. This made our study the largest multi-professional, health workforce survey in the world on this topic.

Of the respondents, half (52%) were aged under 40 years and most (81%) were women, which reflects the predominantly female health workforce in Australia. Most participants were nurses (39%), doctors (31%), or allied health staff (17%) with the remainder working in other health roles. Few healthcare workers (2%) had been infected with COVID-19, but three-quarters (76%) were worried or very worried that their role could lead to them transmitting COVID-19 to their families. The survey found worryingly high levels of psychological distress among healthcare workers during the pandemic. Over half of the healthcare workers who responded to our survey reported significant levels of burnout (71%), severe anxiety (60%), and/or depression (57%). Additionally, many experienced significant changes to social relationships, workplace roles, and finances. More detailed results from the survey, including the demographic and workplace factors associated with mental illness, coping strategies, and organisational change have been published elsewhere.

In addition to measuring mental health, social, financial, and workplace changes, we wanted to understand healthcare workers' experiences, so we included four questions where people could write freely and tell us more. The last question was: "*Is there anything else you want to tell us?*" Normally these are the questions that we all skip over and leave blank in surveys. Yet, once again this survey was unusual as the healthcare workers did not race past these open questions. We received thousands of free-text responses, many of which were long and detailed. Indeed, we received over 250,000 words of heartfelt free text. We read stories of grief, fear, anger, hope, gratitude, and much more. Healthcare workers from every part of the Australian healthcare system shared their personal experiences of, and reflections on, the COVID-19 pandemic and its effect on their families, their work, and their health.

The origins of this book

Some of the healthcare workers who completed our survey expressed little hope that others would ever hear their voices. And indeed, this book was not part of our original research plan. However, as we read the unfiltered emotions and experiences that these healthcare workers offered up to us, we understood that their stories needed to be shared. And it was clear from their responses that healthcare workers wanted other people to hear their words, to understand what they had been through and to bear witness to what they experienced in their work and home lives—both good and bad. These healthcare workers also wanted their narratives and experiences to drive change for the better.

What to expect as you read this book

In this book, we recognise that healthcare workers are the experts in their own lives and that the best way to understand, and learn from their experiences, is to let them speak for themselves. Apart from this introduction, and brief contextual comments introducing each chapter and theme, the words in this book are those of healthcare workers themselves. All of the quotes are free-text responses to the Frontline Healthcare Workers survey, with most drawn from the final question which simply asked: "*Is there anything else you want to tell us?*" Survey responses are grouped by theme, with light editing for clarity and flow. We have provided brief demographic details—profession, area of work, gender, and age range—for each person quoted in this book. Minor details have been changed to protect their anonymity, such as removing the names of hospitals or changing the ages of children.

In compiling this book, we hope to achieve four things. First, to allow healthcare workers to share their stories, and hear from others, as a way of giving words to their experience and finding a sense of shared meaning. Second, we hope to nurture a deeper understanding within the community and among healthcare leaders of how the pandemic affected those providing care. Healthcare workers told us it was sometimes hard to find the words to communicate their experiences with others. We hope that this book will help. Third, we want to shine a light on what these experiences mean for creating a stronger, kinder, and fairer health system for our future. And finally, we wish to create a record of the extraordinary contribution of healthcare workers during the COVID-19 pandemic, as a way of honouring and remembering their contributions.

2

A ROLLER-COASTER OF MOOD AND MEANING

> The Kübler-Ross stages of grief seem to be applicable and I have made my way through all of them. I'm anxious but accepting. I'm scared but competent and confident in my nursing. If I wasn't scared, I would be worried. I empathise with our patients and their families but am mindful keeping myself and my family safe is my priority.
>
> *Nurse, COVID ward, female, age 51–64*

Emotions matter, they make us human. They shape our thoughts, actions, and how we understand and connect with others. The uncertainty and challenges thrown up by the COVID-19 pandemic fuelled a firestorm of emotions among healthcare workers. This chapter presents the array of feelings described by healthcare workers as they navigated the pandemic. As you will read below, healthcare workers felt a full spectrum of emotions, from the positive—enjoying a slower pace of life—to the deeply painful, such as the distress of patients dying and fears for their own lives. The emotional experiences of healthcare workers were complex—changing day-to-day, moment-to-moment, and the depth and breadth of these emotions are evident in the accounts presented here.

Shock

For people around the world, the scale and impact of the pandemic were shocking, and healthcare workers were no different.

> The pandemic caught everyone off guard.
>
> *Allied health practitioner, community care, male, age 51–64*

DOI: 10.4324/9781003228394-2

> Nobody saw it coming.
>
> *Senior doctor, respiratory medicine, male, age 31–40*

> The shock of how the virus is spreading so fast and what I had to do to keep myself and my family safe. Also, seeing some people from my community passing away at my workplace due to this COVID virus. I was stunned.
>
> *Allied health practitioner, intensive care, male, age 31–40*

Some healthcare workers wrote about the unfamiliarity of living or working in a pandemic.

> We are learning as we go. After all, how many of us have lived through a global pandemic?
>
> *Nurse, community care, female, age 51–64*

> This is an unknown, so it's understandable that the support services are not adequate or that people don't know what support they need.
>
> *Pharmacist, general medicine, male, age 31–40*

> Unprecedented times and all that.
>
> *Psychologist, community care, female, age 51–64*

The feeling of shock was sometimes accompanied by a sense of disbelief.

> The pandemic has left a feeling of sadness but also disbelief that it is really happening and has had such a worldwide impact. Surreal really.
>
> *Administrative worker, respiratory medicine, female, age 51–64*

> I often feel a bit numb. Like this is not really happening. Almost like it's a bit of a daze.
>
> *Nurse, medical specialty, female, age 51–64*

Fear

Many healthcare workers described the pandemic as the most frightening experience of their lives.

> I am an emotional wreck working during the pandemic. I am scared every day that I am bringing the virus home to my husband with cancer or my elderly parents. I feel I am unable to support my family emotionally or mentally because I am so scared myself and I spend every day being scared of every patient and being scared for every patient. I am scared of my workmates. I don't have any support and I can't discuss this with my family, and I feel

> completely alone. Any love I did have for the job is gone, and I spend most of my commute to work every day crying.
>
> *Nurse, emergency department, female, age 31–40*

> I have never in my life had the feeling of impending doom and severe anxiety that I experienced in March this year. It felt as if my life, and my family's lives, were at the mercy of a government that did not understand the severity of the pandemic and what was to come.
>
> *Senior doctor, anaesthetics, female, age 41–50*

> Trying to adapt my work—outreach with homeless people—during the pandemic and within restrictions in a way that was safe. Feeling a bit forgotten and unsupported by the organisation. Feeling uncontained, vulnerable, and anxious.
>
> *Nurse, community care, female, age 31–40*

> It was draining, exhausting and frightening.
>
> *Respiratory scientist, female, age 31–40*

> I get scared before shifts.
>
> *Nurse, emergency department, male, age 31–40*

> It's very frightening.
>
> *Social worker, hospital-based, female, age 51–64*

Healthcare workers feared for their own lives and those of their families.

> Unlike soldiers, we didn't enlist to put ourselves at risk for our country; it was a role delegated to us, within the position we were already working so hard in. With the addition of exposing our children and partners to this deadly virus, essentially dragging them to the frontline with us!
>
> *Nurse, emergency department, female, age 31–40*

> We didn't know: Who was coming into the pharmacy? Who may or may not be infected? Some customers were carefree, and you couldn't tell if they practiced social hygiene. It was quite scary to serve some of them who were coughing and wanted help with the cough. We were not wearing masks in the beginning so quite stressful.
>
> *Pharmacist, community care, female, age 31–40*

The anxiety was contagious, with healthcare workers being conscious of the transfer of emotions during clinical interactions with patients.

> Trying to ride the waves of generalised angst, and guard against angst contagion—being based at a "hot" hospital, with patients and staff infected, and hundreds of staff furloughed.
>
> *Psychologist, medical specialty, female, age 41–50*

> I feel very overwhelmed much of the time. I feel like patients are very anxious and they bring that anxiety into consults with me. Everyone is on edge about everything.
>
> *Senior doctor, medical specialty, male, age 31–40*

> While the pandemic may cause significant anxiety in our personal lives, we need to guard against this spreading into our professional lives and interactions with our patients.
>
> *Senior doctor, medical specialty, male, age 41–50*

The fear was felt at work, but also during everyday activities, such as buying food or using public transport. The initial uncertainty about how COVID-19 was spread meant that everyday objects felt like potential sources of contagion.

> In my 23 years of nursing, I have never felt like this. I get anxious going to work and I feel I have to overthink everything I do in order to protect myself and others. There is lots of anxiety and uncertainty amongst colleagues and we are unable to provide the usual support to each other to help during stressful times.
>
> *Nurse, intensive care, female, age 41–50*

> I don't feel safe outside of my home.
>
> *Senior doctor, anaesthetics, female, age 41–50*

> This has taken a toll on me which I was not expecting or prepared for. I feel physically vulnerable and threatened when outside the house. I've previously only felt this way when physically threatened or in a dangerous situation. It feels like everything I do, even collecting groceries or petrol, has a real risk.
>
> *Respiratory scientist, female, age 31–40*

> My concern is that I will catch COVID from a colleague because we are all sharing the space: stair rails, toilets, kettle, keyboards, files.
>
> *Psychologist, outpatient clinic, female, age 41–50*

The fear of death was real.

> The stress at the beginning of the pandemic—waiting for what seemed to be an inevitable wave of death and ill people—felt like standing in front of an oncoming train unable to get off the tracks. Watching the number of dead healthcare workers rising in other countries was horrendous. I located my

will and formulated a document for my parents for "tidying up my affairs" in case I died.

Junior doctor, emergency, female, age 31–40

For the first time ever in my career I felt like my job could seriously harm or even kill me.

Senior doctor, emergency, female, age 31–40

I have nights when I lie awake and I worry that I will get sick and die. I have had discussions with my older children and told them what I would like to happen to my body should I die, but I am also feeling optimistic that all will be well eventually. I usually stress more after I have had prolonged exposure to a COVID-positive patient who has been extremely unwell, and I have been in the room with them for up to six hours in PPE.

Nurse, emergency department, female, age 41–50

Huge anxiety. Sleepless nights. I wrote a will to identify who was going to look after my 11-month-old baby if my husband and I both died.

Senior doctor, emergency department, female, age 31–40

I wrote a will this year. I really should have had one already, but a lot of nurses are now dead, so I wrote one.

Nurse, emergency department, male, age 31–40

Fear is an emotion that helps us to identify threats and motivates us to avoid danger. Some healthcare workers emphasised that their anxiety was not pathological, but rather proportionate to the threat they were facing.

People that work in hospitals are not stupid. A weekly meditation session or some daft PowerPoint presentation is not going to convince frontline staff that their anxiety is not justified.

Allied health practitioner, community care, female, age 31–40

The best remedy for COVID-19 anxiety is the numbers coming down!

Senior doctor, medical specialty, female, age 41–50

I've been watching the COVID case numbers and related deaths each day—dread them but can't stop reading them.

Nurse, palliative care, female, age 51–64

I'm due for another asymptomatic screening test this week and I do feel myself a bit more anxious waiting for the result, but increased relief when a test is negative. That relieves my anxiety for a bit.

Senior doctor, general medicine, female, age 41–50

Anticipation

Many healthcare workers were apprehensive that the worst was yet to come.

> COVID has added a layer of strain and apprehension that can exacerbate the day to day challenges of my role.
>
> *Allied health assistant, surgical, male, age 41–50*

> Apprehensions, not knowing when and how bad it could get. Not knowing if you or a family member might get sick and what the outcomes could be.
>
> *Junior doctor, hospital aged care, female, age 20–30*

> This isn't just a bad day or two at work—it is a sustained period of fear, increased workload and trauma and I am concerned about what the ongoing impacts of this will be.
>
> *Nurse, community care, female, age 41–50*

> While every effort is made to ensure that we as health care workers are supported, I fear for the general community and the ramifications to society for the future.
>
> *Nurse, pathology, female, age 51–64*

> While COVID is happening people may seem to be managing fine, and do, but the aftermath will be worrying.
>
> *Occupational therapist, medical specialty, female, age 31–40*

The anticipation of future health issues focused on three main areas: mental illness, long-COVID, and patient care. The first area of concern was the risk of post-traumatic stress disorder (PTSD) and mental health difficulties among healthcare workers.

> I'm feeling at my worst only now that the worst of this wave is easing. I'm surprised that it has hit me afterwards and it upsets me when I look back at what we did.
>
> *Nurse, intensive care, female, age 31–40*

> As a nurse educator, I have seen a lot of staff suffering the beginnings of PTSD and I believe this will have a flow-on effect long term.
>
> *Nurse, respiratory medicine, female, age 31–40*

> I fear finishing it all with PTSD.
>
> *Senior doctor, emergency medicine, male, age 41–50*

> I'm scared of the long-term effect of COVID-19 on my mental health and professional identity as a nurse. I'm finding it hard to distinguish burnout from

> PTSD symptoms. I fear that the long journey in recovering from COVID will impact my mental health more negatively.
>
> *Nurse, emergency department, female, age 20–30*

The second area of apprehension related to the possible—and still unknown—long-term consequences of infection with COVID-19.

> Being aware of the longer-term issues possible with COVID causes worry!
>
> *Senior doctor, medical specialty, male, age 51–64*

> The long-term effects of COVID-19 on lungs, kidneys, hearts, and brains may be a major challenge for health systems in the future. This does not seem to be getting much attention yet.
>
> *Senior doctor, respiratory medicine, male, age 31–40*

And as we show in more detail in Chapter 13, healthcare workers also worried about the long-term consequences of the pandemic restrictions for patient care, rates of mental illness in the general population, and quality of life.

> I keep thinking about all the people (non-COVID patients) who will have long-term impacts on their health due to the reduced level of care/therapy they have received during the pandemic. Thinking about the toll on our system into the future stresses me out.
>
> *Speech pathologist, general medicine, male, age 20–30*

> Allied health—dental, physiotherapy, psychology etc—are about to be overwhelmed and there needs to be long-term investment in these areas to meet people's ongoing needs after COVID. Waitlists for public care have blown out and will have ongoing effects for years to come.
>
> *Allied health practitioner, emergency dental, female, age 20–30*

Some workers expressed concern about the capacity of the mental health system to cope with this anticipated increase in demand.

> Mental health will have a long tail once we are out of lockdown and I am worried that there won't be sufficient supports at the community level to support people in this extraordinary time.
>
> *Psychologist, community care, female, age 51–64*

> As the mental health fallout from the pandemic is likely to continue for many years, the wellbeing of the frontline health staff will be of utmost importance to avoid mass burnout.
>
> *Psychologist, community care, female, age 51–64*

> While I feel positive about the care we give overall, the burden and impact on us will take a long time to recover from. And we will soon need to treat the people affected by the economic downturn that has started—the homeless, the unemployed. So, the next wave is looming.
>
> *Nurse, medical specialty, female, age 51–64*

Sadness

Sadness was a common emotion, with healthcare workers describing low mood and tearfulness.

> Overwhelming sadness.
>
> *Speech pathologist, hospital aged care, female, age 31–40*

> I have often started crying for little apparent reason.
>
> *Senior doctor, anaesthetics, male, age 51–64*

> Feeling teary and emotional in response to news stories about situations of suffering.
>
> *Senior doctor, medical specialty, male, age 51–64*

Some experienced a lack of motivation and loss of pleasure in previously enjoyable activities.

> The impact of COVID 19 worsened during my annual leave. I couldn't find interest in any indoor activities, but also wasn't very motivated to study.
>
> *Junior doctor, surgical, female, age 20–30*

> I have great plans to do things like online yoga, but then the days come and go, and I don't do it. Lack of motivation, even though I know it would be good for me. I'm not even enjoying Zoom happy hours/catch ups with friends any more—there's nothing to talk about except the virus which just gets me down more. I'm normally a positive, energetic person and am hating the way I feel now.
>
> *Physiotherapist, emergency department, female, age 51–64*

> Life is boring in lock down. It is very hard to be motivated to work with no rewards. No holidays, no shopping, no travel.
>
> *Senior doctor, emergency department, female, age 51–64*

They also wrote about feelings of hopelessness and despair.

> It's hard to stay positive and encourage other staff members when you are tired.
>
> *Hospital cleaner, female, age 51–64*

> The second lockdown has completely broken my spirit. I have little motivation for life and I feel like all the hard work isn't making a difference anymore.
>
> *Administrative worker, medical specialty, female, age 20–30*

> General flat demeanor. No-one has any forward or future thoughts, not even a chat about a future holiday because that just is senseless.
>
> *Radiographer, emergency department, female, age 51–64*

> Feeling defeated.
>
> *Radiographer, emergency department, female, age 20–30*

As we show in Chapter 8, healthcare workers described being burnt out, and the associated shifts in their emotional responses.

> I'm burnt out. The impact of COVID has affected my empathy. I feel like best practice is unachievable and that there are so many barriers to providing care.
>
> *Physiotherapist, general medicine, female, age 31–40*

> There have been very varied responses from health care workers. Some have only thought about themselves and others have stepped up and taken on other roles. I feel I have become a bit jaded and judgmental. I hope my attitude will return to normal.
>
> *Occupational therapist, medical specialty, female, age 51–64*

> If I make it through this with my humanity intact, I will be stunned.
>
> *Medical scientist, medical specialty, female, age 51–64*

The level of distress felt by some healthcare workers was overwhelming, particularly for those with existing mental health issues.

> The depression I was diagnosed with before the pandemic hit, has unfortunately completely spiraled out of control to the point of suicidality.
>
> *Junior doctor, emergency department, female, age 31–40*

Some healthcare workers—particularly those working in aged care settings where the majority of deaths occurred—felt alone with their despair, unwilling to burden others with their grief and unable to adequately communicate the reality of their days.

> I have cried every day for two months since the nursing home outbreaks have begun. I have been unable to speak with family or friends about my work without crying. I have not even been able to talk to other doctors, as they have not experienced the same things I have. Because of all of this, I have not spoken to my friends for two months. My children have become extremely

> distressed and anxious because of my emotional distress and because of my enormous workload … I have worked hard and with minimal support over my career as a doctor. BUT I have never worked this hard or experienced this degree of stress or emotional toll from the work I have been doing the last two months. During the height of the pandemic, I had hoped I would get COVID so I would not have to come to work.
>
> *Senior doctor, residential aged care, female, age 41–50*

Many others just wanted the pandemic to be over.

> I am feeling worn down by the need for vigilance and the erosion of relationships. I'm worried that we will not see a return to "normal" life. I'm struggling to keep a positive attitude. I want to crawl into a cave and hide until this is all over.
>
> *Psychologist, community care, female, age 51–64*

> It's shit. I've had enough and I want it to go away please.
>
> *Nurse, emergency department, male, age 31–40*

> I feel absolutely drained, I want to go to sleep and wake up when it's over, I'm so, so over it that I feel I am further isolating myself because I just don't want to think about it.
>
> *Nurse, emergency department, female, age 31–40*

> If I hadn't been able to talk to friends that just happened to be online when I was locked up in Sydney, I would've jumped out the window (except it wouldn't open) just to make it all stop.
>
> *Senior doctor, radiology, male, age 41–50*

Guilt

Healthcare workers described feelings of guilt because they felt unable to do enough for their colleagues, patients, families, and communities.

> It's difficult for those outside healthcare work to understand the feelings/emotions. I often feel guilty that I can't do more.
>
> *Nurse, perioperative care, female, age 41–50*

> I feel guilty that I am not pulling my weight as I do not have face-to-face contact with patients. I know in my mind this is not true, but it still sits there.
>
> *Nurse, community care, female, age 51–64*

> I do feel a small degree of guilt for not directly contributing to managing the pandemic and not feeling like I'm "doing my part" so to speak.
>
> *Junior doctor, surgical, male, age 20–30*

> Not being able to help more due to pregnancy has caused feelings of frustration and guilt about not being able to help colleagues.
>
> *General practitioner, female, age 31–40*

Anger

Healthcare workers also wrote about their anger, ranging from day-to-day grumpiness and frustration through to unexpected rage.

> I just feel so irritated with everyone and everything.
>
> *Administrative worker, medical specialty, female, age 20–30*

> I'm overreacting to situations that normally would not bother me.
>
> *Nurse, medical specialty, female, age 51–64*

> I feel angry at the lockdown. I feel that it is so unfair and the longest around the world. I feel more reckless than usual, I am doing anything to just get through but the longer the pandemic plays out, and the longer my ward has restrictions, the more hopeless and angry I feel.
>
> *Nurse, general medicine, female, age 20–30*

Common precipitants of anger and frustration were increased care responsibilities at home, ill-informed members of the public, and inadequate protections at work. The frustration of childcare and home-schooling was a common theme among healthcare workers with children.

> When I arrived home, I started home-school with my daughter, we are all trying our best to juggle work and home-school in this pandemic. All of a sudden, my anger and frustration took hold of me. If I could have thrown the laptop, I certainly would have! I felt really down after that incident. I didn't seek professional help, I just stopped doing home-school for four days and then I was fine to go back to work.
>
> *Nurse, hospital aged care, female, age 20–30*

For other healthcare workers, their frustration was sparked by people who claimed to know more than the experts, and who disputed the seriousness of the disease or the need for restrictive public health measures.

> I have become hugely irritated by the outliers and the armchair "epidemiologists".
>
> *General practitioner, female, age 71+*

> Not useful when self-proclaimed experts give their opinion on how the pandemic should be managed despite not having appropriate experience, data, or knowledge.
>
> *Senior doctor, respiratory medicine, female, age 31–40*

> Disappointment with people who think government measures are too harsh. I have difficulty dealing with people who think COVID is fake.
>
> *Nurse, perioperative care, female, age 41–50*

> I would like to see that people understand the severity of the situation and respond accordingly instead of refusing to accept the reality and not doing their part to get things better for everyone.
>
> *Disability support worker, hospital aged care, male, age 51–64*

> To hear about people who deny the existence of the disease makes me really angry for families who have lost people to COVID and who were (more than likely) unable to be with them when they died. Especially as a nurse who has palliated COVID patients who have died without their families beside them. That's the saddest situation I've ever seen as a nurse in my 11 years.
>
> *Nurse, intensive care, female, age 31–40*

> I find it EXTREMELY frustrating hearing people deny the existence of COVID or downplay the disease. I have held the hands of a dying woman as she passed away from COVID.
>
> *Nurse, intensive care, female age 20–30*

As we explore in more detail in later chapters, healthcare workers also expressed anger at those leaders and organisations who failed to keep them safe.

> Currently, if a hospital was a building site no-one would be allowed to enter as it would be deemed unsafe. But healthcare workers are expected to turn up and keep going with rationed PPE. How shocking is that!
>
> *Nurse, emergency department, female, age 41–50*

> I think because I'm in a metropolitan public hospital looking after COVID patients, I really found the initial "denial" of workplace transmission in healthcare settings rage-inducing. I have colleagues who clearly caught COVID at work and I don't appreciate the gaslighting of healthcare workers who fall ill.
>
> *Senior doctor, general medicine, female, age 41–50*

> I was so angry when a colleague was threatened to be stood down for asking for a N95 mask.
>
> *Senior doctor, general medicine, female, age 41–50*

Disgust

Feelings of aversion, or the even stronger emotion of disgust, were expressed towards people who flaunted precautions that had been put in place to save lives.

I am appalled at the lack of care of members of our community who have kept the virus going by exercising their "rights" at the expense of others.

Social worker, intensive care and palliative care, female, age 31–40

All these people who flaunt the rules, refuse to take precautions, and exploit "freedom of speech" to vocalise misinformation and harm others. I want these people to care for a COVID patient without PPE seeing as they don't believe in it—so I don't have to. It's a slap in the face of someone who risks their health and the lives of their family every day, when you have so many disrespectful and apathetic members of society who are so selfish that they believe their lives are more valuable than others. And if they get COVID they would expect to be treated in a hospital, wouldn't they? If it was their child intubated in a bed struggling to breathe, they'd want the highest level of medical care, wouldn't they? Even when they were the ones knowingly non-compliant with basic precautions. They can stay home and stay safe. But we can't stay home.

Nurse, intensive care, female, age 20–30

It's frustrating seeing people break the rules and put us all backwards but blame healthcare workers for being in cluster outbreaks. The attitude needs to change.

Allied health assistant, medical specialty, female, age 20–30

As a healthcare worker it is so hard having to listen to the Melbourne protestors with their anti-vaccination, anti-mask, anti-lockdown attitudes, while my husband and I—who are both healthcare workers—and all my colleagues are working so hard and sacrificing a lot to get through this. The selfish attitudes, ignorance, the way some people just don't care if vulnerable members of our community suffer, has been confronting and upsetting, when caring is what we do every day.

Nurse, medical specialty, female, age 41–50

I have lost three close colleagues I worked with here and abroad, directly due to COVID. Watching all these people doing silly riots, and their deviant attitudes to police when asked for their details, is a slap in healthcare workers' faces.

Nurse, mental health, male, age 31–40

I wish that some people would see us as part of the solution and wouldn't see us as part of the problem e.g., antivaxxers, COVID conspiracy believers, or herd immunity supporters. Their evangelistic beliefs don't need to be targeted at health professionals.

Allied health practitioner, community care, male, age 51–64

> The pandemic has brought out the true colours of people. They are either amazing or truly selfish.
>
> *Administrative worker, emergency department, female, age 41–50*

Serenity

One positive feature of the pandemic was the chance for some healthcare workers to slow down and live a simpler life.

> COVID has made me think twice about life in a positive way. Going back to the basics and not living a fast-paced life. It has actually been a helpful thing for me.
>
> *Administrative worker, female, age 41–50*

> The first lockdown I quite enjoyed. It was a unique chance to slow down and see how an alternate life could be lived.
>
> *Administrative worker, medical specialty, female, age 20–30*

> We have all slowed down and appreciate each other more.
>
> *Physiotherapist, surgical, female, age 20–30*

> I have enjoyed the slower pace of life—less traffic, less noise, more cyclists, getting to know all the river walks near my house, connecting with friends.
>
> *Occupational therapist, community care, female, age 51–64*

> It has been helpful to reflect on purpose at work, connect with colleagues, play with kids or do something with them depending on age (cooking, board games, learn a language, extended dinner time for talking about the day), play with friends—online movies, board games, dancing, walking.
>
> *General practitioner, male, age 51–64*

For some, the calmer pace of life, imposed by the lockdown, brought them closer to friends and family.

> I have had more time with my family because I haven't been quite as busy as normal so this aspect has been positive.
>
> *Senior doctor, respiratory medicine, male, age 51–64*

> I have become closer to my children and more involved with what happens with schooling. Improved routine at home, back to the basics of life without pressures and expectations from communities and sporting activities.
>
> *Nurse, emergency department, female, age 41–50*

Several healthcare workers expressed a hope that they would be able to hold onto these feelings after the pandemic ended.

> I hope the importance and benefits of exercise and sleep, the luxury of breathing and face-to-face interactions, are never taken for granted again.
>
> *Respiratory scientist, female, age 31–40*

> I don't want to be stressed or go back to the way my work was before COVID—I didn't realise how stressed I was prior to lockdown. Life is more peaceful now in some ways.
>
> *Nurse, general medicine, female, age 51–64*

Admiration

Healthcare workers expressed appreciation for colleagues and for the support of the wider community.

> People are amazing.
>
> *Senior doctor, private practice, female, age 51–64*

This appreciation was most commonly directed towards colleagues.

> My colleagues have been truly amazing and resilient throughout this whole situation. I have nothing but respect and love for how hard everyone has been working and how strong they all are.
>
> *Nurse, hospital aged care, female, age 31–40*

> I admire the healthcare workers that provide endless support to the sick and elderly in nursing homes.
>
> *Allied health practitioner, medical specialty, female, age 65–70*

> I think that all healthcare staff are doing an amazing job considering the circumstances they are under. I believe we are all learning about how resilient we are and how life is so precious.
>
> *Administrative worker, community care, female, age 41–50*

As we hear in Chapter 15, healthcare workers also expressed appreciation for the community support they had received.

> I feel proud of the resilience. Many people have had to rise above and provide "paying forward" moments. Like that extra care for someone battling, leaving flowers for the girls at the hospital cafe, or money for a coffee for the next patron.
>
> *Administrative worker, medical specialty, female, age 65–70*

> I have really appreciated the little things—occasional small gifts, acts of kindness of others.
>
> *Senior doctor, hospital aged care, female, age 41–50*

Changing and uncertain emotions

Healthcare workers' emotional journeys were rarely linear. Many experienced different emotions on different days—or even within the space of a single day—from the highs of cohesion and contribution, to despair and disillusionment, through to hope and reconstruction.

> It's a bit of a roller-coaster of mood and sense of self and meaning.
>
> *Occupational therapist, community care, female, age 51–64*

> My emotional state fluctuates. I often hold it together, but there are days when it's overwhelming.
>
> *Senior doctor, medical specialty, female, age 51–64*

> It is a dynamic situation and a person feels different emotions at the same time. It's not easy to put in writing.
>
> *Senior doctor, intensive care, male, age 41–50*

> It's a tough situation and everyone is doing their best to get through it.
>
> *Nurse, palliative care, female, age 31–40*

> We have all had different and constantly changing levels of optimism throughout the pandemic. We are all doing our best to keep each other afloat depending on how much energy we each have on any given day.
>
> *Nurse, surgical, female, age 20–30*

Some felt an obligation to appear calm and positive around children, colleagues, or patients.

> When in conversation with colleagues and direct management I felt I needed to be "strong", but then I get home and feel weak. I struggled to let the people at work know how hard it is.
>
> *Pharmacist, general medicine, male, age 31–40*

Others experienced new—and at times overwhelming—emotional responses, with the stresses of the pandemic pushing them outside of their own personal "window of tolerance" within which emotions could be regulated.

> I generally think I'm doing fine, but I will have sudden switches in emotional state. I've noticed I become more emotional than I usually would about a

sad event—almost daily—then go back to "normal". I also find some things inappropriately humorous—more than normal.

Respiratory scientist, female, age 31–40

Some healthcare workers found it difficult to even find the words to describe their emotions.

It's hard to quantify how you feel in such strange times.

Nurse, female, age 51–64

Hindsight will be a time of reflection. Whilst we are in the midst of this pandemic, we are just running with the evolving goalposts.

Administrative worker, community care, female, age 51–64

Ask me when the pandemic is over, I'm just in survival mode currently.

Nurse, medical specialty, female, age 31–40

Even filling this out has brought tears to my eyes so maybe I'm not coping as well as I thought I was.

Nurse, intensive care, female, age 51–64

3

PERVASIVE, PRECARIOUS, AND PERILOUS

> People working in frontline healthcare, who are trying to do their best in a rapidly changing landscape, are also impacted by effects on family, home-schooling, elderly relatives, and basic day-to-day issues. The pandemic affects every aspect of our lives and is impossible to get away from. I have a brief moment when I wake up—until I realise the pandemic is still here—which is not invaded by the pandemic, but it is constantly in my mind.
>
> *Senior doctor, hospital aged care, female, age 41–50*

The COVID-19 pandemic was constant and inescapable in the lives of healthcare workers. While they recognised the pandemic was difficult for everyone, they also spoke about the unique challenges and stresses experienced by those providing patient care. Healthcare workers are normally seen as resilient and adaptable in the face of stressful events. However, the pervasiveness of the pandemic at home, in the media, and in an increasingly challenging workplace, meant there was no respite. In this chapter, we hear about healthcare workers feeling unable to escape the pandemic, being constantly worried about infecting others, and facing financial insecurity and uncertainty about the future. Healthcare workers also worried about the tensions between stringent lockdown restrictions and individual, social, and economic wellbeing.

The pervasiveness of COVID-19 in daily life

The pandemic was ever-present in the everyday lives of healthcare workers. They were working as professionals caring for people affected by the pandemic and living as members of the community experiencing the pandemic, at the same time.

DOI: 10.4324/9781003228394-3

> As a psychologist working in a pandemic, I am also a person living in a pandemic. There is a strange sharing of experience with my patients that can be helpful but also means I need to focus on a patient's experience rather than assuming that it's like my own. Just another complexity to manage in the work.
>
> *Psychologist, mental health, female, age 51–64*

> Although we are health staff, we are also the community members we claim to be serving. We have the same fears and worries about the impact of COVID on ourselves and our families regardless of our training or the fact that we are professionals.
>
> *Social worker, community care, male, age 41–50*

The multi-layered stressors of being a healthcare worker, providing patient care in a pandemic, and being an everyday citizen living in a pandemic, were impossible to disentangle.

> This has been a unique time and a challenge for everyone. As a healthcare worker I have always been aware of, and looked after, my physical and mental health. However, since March there has been unprecedented stress in the workplace, at home, and in society changing how we live which has certainly affected my energy levels and mood. I think we need to remember that healthcare workers have not only dealt with huge change and stress at work, but also in their personal lives.
>
> *Physiotherapist, community care, female, age 31–40*

> It has been difficult to separate the effects of the pandemic on my work and home life independently, as they impact each other. I felt very concerned for my colleagues with limited social supports, financial stability, and trauma histories. Particularly those who were furloughed.
>
> *Social worker, hospital aged care, female, age 31–40*

> The impact of COVID is so enduring and widespread that it is impossible to distract yourself from thinking about it for large periods of the day. Especially when you are constantly reminded of it. You're in PPE all day at work, you get temperature checks and questionnaires everywhere you go, you have a curfew to abide by. You hear it on the news, your friends are on Zoom, you can't visit your family interstate or overseas. It's just constant for weeks and months on end. The psychological and social impacts from the restrictions are so immense that they have contributed enormous harms to our community.
>
> *Junior doctor, anaesthetics, male, age 20–30*

> Our home lives are still stressful when we get home from stressful days.
>
> *Nurse, palliative care, female, age 41–50*

> Never getting a break—you are always living it. Work is stressful, you go home, live a mediocre COVID-allowed life, and repeat.
>
> *Nurse, emergency department, male, age 20–30*

> I feel like I can't go anywhere to relax. I can't escape. I'm stressed at home, stressed at work. And working in an emergency department, it's stressful at baseline.
>
> *Nurse, emergency department, female, age 20–30*

> The pandemic just produces a baseline stress level that is constantly in the back of your mind.
>
> *Physiotherapist, intensive care, female, age 20–30*

While working in healthcare was a constant reminder of COVID-19, healthcare workers also reported that the pandemic was impossible to escape from because of the infiltration of "COVID-19 talk" into every part of their lives, from their social networks to news and social media platforms. Some healthcare workers placed boundaries around their use of social and traditional media to provide some shelter from the constant barrage of news and debate about COVID-19.

> The hardest part is talking about it all the time. At least people at home can escape it a bit. Then all of social media is arguments about it.
>
> *Nurse, emergency department, female, age 41–50*

> It is currently gruelling and relentless. It is exacerbated by the fact that there is no escape from work, as you get home and COVID is plastered across the media.
>
> *Pharmacist, female, age 20–30*

> It's hard to escape sometimes. Leave work and it is all over the news, social media, and in every everyday conversation. It is exhausting.
>
> *Nurse, intensive care, female, age 31–40*

> The constant bombarding of COVID-19 on all media and social platforms decreases the ability to switch off and remove oneself from being involved when they are not working.
>
> *Paramedic, male, age 31–40*

> The dilemma of following the media has frustrated me. On the one hand, I want to be as well informed as possible and keep up to date with latest developments. On the other hand, I'm sick to death of hearing about COVID, COVID, COVID.
>
> *Nurse, community care, male, age 51–64*

> The best thing I have done is snooze all the news outlets and friends/family that do nothing but talk about COVID!
>
> *Social worker, acute care, female, age 41–50*

> Decreasing my exposure to the media coverage of it and the social media apps, which would highlight a lot of radical and seemingly biased views, really helped me find the opportunity to unwind, detox from the pandemic and just enjoy the time in lockdown as some personal private time.
>
> *Nurse, infectious diseases, female, age 20–30*

> I know we are all doing our best but it's exhausting. Not tuning into the media regularly helps to focus on what needs to be done and not thinking about what I can't control.
>
> *Nurse, general medicine, female, age 41–50*

> The media onslaught does not assist with relaxation post-work but sharing social media memes with friends and family have kept me sane.
>
> *Senior doctor, emergency department, female, age 41–50*

> I think social media has been the worst enemy throughout COVID. As an educator I've encouraged staff to not read and not get involved but I have found myself using it and getting angry at all the different theories and politics surrounding COVID and rarely about the general health side of things.
>
> *Nurse, education, female, age 31–40*

Constant anxiety and worry

Health professionals shared similar anxieties about the pandemic as many others in the community, but their fears were amplified by working in a high-risk setting. Many shared their worries about infecting vulnerable others, especially their partners, family members, friends, and patients.

> My biggest problem is how to safeguard my family from the risky job I do.
>
> *Junior doctor, emergency department, male, age 51–64*

> I have three frontline healthcare workers in my household. This worries me. It increases the potential for this to get into my home and once one of us gets it, it will be hard to prevent the rest from getting it.
>
> *Senior doctor, emergency department, male, age 51–64*

> I am not wanting my COVID work and high-risk face-to-face exposure to affect my family physically and emotionally.
>
> *Psychologist, community care, male, age 51–64*

> I live with my partner, and although I am extremely careful my biggest anxiety is around her catching COVID and knowing it most likely will have come from me.
>
> *Student, infectious diseases, female, age 20–30*

> I'm worried about the implications for my family if I contract COVID. We live in a very small unit without outdoor space. I have an 18-month-old. It will be almost impossible to isolate from him and my husband in our home.
>
> *Junior doctor, hospital aged care, female, age 31–40*

> I am returning to work soon and now am feeling anxious about feeling underprepared with dealing with potential COVID-19 patients. I am also worried about passing on the disease to my young children at home.
>
> *Junior doctor, medical specialty, female, age 31–40*

> My work concerns are minor. My major concern is ensuring I do not bring the infection home to my husband, otherwise, it's a normal day in ICU.
>
> *Nurse, intensive care, female, age 51–64*

> The fear of transmitting the virus to household members with underlying health conditions is exhausting at times. The worst part is that there is no end date.
>
> *Nurse, residential aged care, female, age 51–64*

> I know that if my family gets COVID, it will most likely be from ME giving it to them as I care for COVID patients at least two to three times a week.
>
> *Nurse, intensive care, female, age 20–30*

The worry about infecting others meant healthcare workers took steps to reduce the risk, but this often came at an emotional cost.

> I lived apart from my husband because of his lung disease and had no physical contact and this took its toll on me.
>
> *Nurse, respiratory medicine, female, age 51–64*

> I never saw my grandchildren even when the restrictions lessened because I was concerned if I contracted it, I would pass it on.
>
> *Nurse, community care, female, age 51–64*

> My elderly neighbours understand that I can't help them as much, but other friends and family do not understand that I have been self-isolating more outside of work to prevent the risk of spreading any infection to them and their families.
>
> *Podiatrist, community care, female, age 31–40*

> It was hard to explain to family and friends why I was so anxious about becoming an unwitting carrier. It was difficult for them to understand how much my work had changed, and why I was overwhelmed trying to make seemingly simple choices. It was difficult to explain the impact of constant hypervigilance at work and not be frustrated when they weren't taking it as seriously.
>
> *Occupational therapist, community care, female, age 31–40*

Healthcare workers are also worried about the danger of unwittingly infecting their patients.

> There is a level of anxiety we are all carrying consistently, with the fear that we will be the source of an outbreak. To be honest this is my greatest stress.
>
> *Social worker, palliative care, female, age 31–40*

> My greatest stress is giving it to a vulnerable patient. Every time I treat someone, I worry about them dying if they get it from me. I am healthy and think I will be okay if I get it, but if I gave it to someone, I couldn't forgive myself.
>
> *Physiotherapist, community care, female, age 41–50*

> I worry one of us will bring it into the facility and our patients will die.
>
> *Nurse, hospital aged care, female, age 65–70*

> The concern being my patients who are immunocompromised and what COVID might do to them.
>
> *Nurse, emergency department, female, age 31–40*

> Healthcare workers are also afraid of bringing the virus into vulnerable patient groups, not just contracting it themselves.
>
> *Speech pathologist, hospital aged care, female, age 41–50*

To reduce the risk they posed to vulnerable family members, some healthcare workers made financial sacrifices, took additional leave, or changed their place of work.

> I was on maternity leave when the pandemic kicked off. My other half is also a junior doctor. I ended up staying on maternity leave longer as we were concerned about having at least one parent at home who wasn't exposed.
>
> *Junior doctor, intensive care, female, age 31–40*

> I tried to work on a COVID ward but my anxiety for the well-being of my family meant I couldn't do more than one shift. I was too stressed. I would like to contribute to the pandemic workforce, but my family comes first. I am sorry for this.
>
> *Senior doctor, surgical, female, age 41–50*

Financial insecurities and precarious work

Healthcare workers also wrote about financial insecurity and uncertainty. Along with many others in the community, some healthcare workers experienced real or potential loss of income and faced difficult financial choices.

> I work casually to add to my income. However due to the pandemic, I preferred not to pick up extra work because of the fear that I will expose myself and my family to a risk of bringing COVID into my household. I have family members who are vulnerable.
>
> *Nurse, administration, female, age 41–50*

Concerns about precarious employment and financial insecurity were particularly notable among those with less control over their work and with lower-paid jobs: casual workers, private contractors, students, and the self-employed. These groups suffered financial consequences if their workplace closed or reduced their hours, or if they were furloughed after being exposed to the virus. If they didn't work, they didn't earn.

> If I don't go to work, I don't get paid.
>
> *Administrative worker, community care, female, age 31–40*

> Time off work means no income. No income increases stress.
>
> *Nurse, palliative care, female, age 51–64*

> I have cancer and started chemo around the same time as the second wave so have been unable to work in my usual area, which has been the main COVID ward, due to being immunocompromised. I feel like I shouldn't lose income just because unfortunate circumstances prevent me from working.
>
> *Nurse, infectious diseases, female, age 51–64*

> International students had a lot of struggles with finances and even covering basic needs. I'm not expecting students to get the same treatment as staff, nor should we, but some acknowledgement and provision of information would have been nice. Many of these issues are not even under the scope of the hospital executives or the health department, but I just want to highlight some of the unique challenges that students had during this pandemic.
>
> *Student, palliative care, female, age 20–30*

> As a student, and part-time employee, I wasn't eligible for JobKeeper. This was financially incredibly stressful as I live out of home and have to pay my own rent. It was an incredibly stressful time, with no flexibility on the university's behalf.
>
> *Student, intensive care, female, age 20–30*

With restrictions to many health service activities (e.g., elective surgery), health practitioners working in private practice reported decreased income and increased costs.

> I have had a 40 percent drop in income due to loss of private earnings.
>
> *Senior doctor, anaesthetics, male, age 31–40*

> Billings have been affected meaning longer hours at work with little reward. This is scarcely sustainable and adds additional worry to already stretched practitioners.
>
> *General practitioner, female, age 41–50*

> There has been very little to no support for GP practices. Enforced bulk-billing [inability to charge a fee on top of the government rebate] was a dreadful thing to impose on practices when we were already faced with increased costs associated with infection control. To amplify the financial stress, many practices saw a reduction in patients presenting and therefore a reduction in income.
>
> *General practitioner, female, age 41–50*

> Loss of income for contractors when taking time off for illness and swabs is extremely difficult. Self-education on your own time and dime is exhausting. Increased costs to practices have threatened the viability of primary care.
>
> *General practitioner, female, age 51–64*

> Doctors in private practice especially have no JobKeeper, no guarantee of regular work if the surgeon is sick, or cases are cancelled due to COVID. There is no support system.
>
> *Senior doctor, anaesthetics, female, age 41–50*

Other healthcare workers wrote about their experiences of insecure housing or the financial burden of self-funding their own accommodation to self-isolate away from their household members.

> I would have felt more supported if I was offered isolation accommodation while I was working in the COVID [screening] clinic. Instead, I bore the financial cost of renting a motel for a month to protect my family.
>
> *Junior doctor, medical specialty, female, age 20–30*

> I was furloughed for two weeks, and had to move into an apartment temporarily, to not affect my family who were very worried that I could be detrimental to their health. They tried to hide it, but I could just tell. As such, I didn't have proper cooking utensils, a small fridge, poor storage etc, and could not go to the shops. I relied on people to bring me shopping, to get it

> delivered. Yes, I was getting paid, but my expenses went up exponentially, and I am now spending over three times more than what I normally would. Support financially for things like this need to be taken into account for the future. It just adds that extra element of mental stress and anxiety over finances.
>
> *Pharmacist, general medicine, male, age 31–40*

> I am completely unwilling to risk bringing COVID home to my family so I will have to personally pay for a hotel if I'm in that situation. It would be great to give healthcare workers more support to protect their families.
>
> *Junior doctor, medical specialty, female, age 31–40*

> Difficulty balancing self-interests and public health interests during this global pandemic. My fiancé and I have remained physically isolated from each other due to having direct contact with COVID patients at two different health services. This is a sacrifice that has been difficult mentally and affects us financially.
>
> *Junior doctor, female, age 20–30*

> I rent with friends. Because of the COVID pandemic my living situation has changed five times. The changes have been due to unreliable income for one housemate meaning he had to move out, a landlord selling our house, housemates being deployed to work in different areas. My housemates are like my family and thus so much change has taken a real toll on my resilience and anxiety.
>
> *Nurse, intensive care, female, age 51–64*

Several healthcare workers believed that the government should have done more to provide financial security for healthcare workers during the pandemic.

> Financial support must be an absolute priority. If more people had financial security, I think the mental health problems would be significantly reduced.
>
> *Student, general medicine, female, age 20–30*

Another group of healthcare workers reported struggling financially because their partners or other household members had lost their jobs and/or livelihoods.

> My husband's small business has been adversely affected so he has done most of the home-schooling, and I have worked a bit more than usual, so we are financially okay.
>
> *Senior doctor, general medicine, female, age 41–50*

> The hardest thing was watching family members go through financial ruin from lockdown restrictions and trying to aid a little financially, but not being able to support them enough.
>
> *Senior doctor, female, age 31–40*

> We put the mortgage on hold as my husband had to close down his café.
>
> *Nurse, emergency department, female, age 41–50*

> My partner is not working. We are struggling to pay the bills.
>
> *Administrative worker medical specialty, female, age 20–30*

> My partner lost his job due to the pandemic and he has not been paid any allowance from the government, and the loss of income has deeply affected us.
>
> *Nursing, general medicine, female, age 20–30*

> COVID-19 has ruined our way of life that we lived previous to this pandemic. Many businesses and individuals have lost income and people are basically over it and want to be normal again. I want things to be normal again.
>
> *Nurse, community care, female, age 51–64*

Weighing up the benefits and the risks of lockdown

Throughout their responses, healthcare workers wrote about the pervasiveness of pandemic-related restrictions, and reflected on the real and potential harms posed by lockdown. Most healthcare workers agreed with the necessity of restrictions to protect the health of communities, while recognising that these restrictions came at a significant cost.

> The lockdowns are necessary but are a major impediment to living a happy life.
>
> *Senior doctor, emergency department, male, age 51–64*

Some healthcare workers questioned whether the harms caused by the stringent lockdown restrictions might eventually outweigh the benefits.

> The psychosocial impact of lockdown has been troubling and I wonder whether it was worth it on balance?
>
> *Physiotherapist, community care, female, age 41–50*

> Isolation. Lockdown without hope. Just a hope that a vaccine will be found. Otherwise this strategy does not seem to have an endpoint.
>
> *Junior doctor, emergency department, male, age 31-40*

> I feel that there is an enormous cost to lockdown that does not receive the front-page attention of COVID deaths and will have a far greater impact on health and wellbeing than COVID. I find it frustrating that the government and media are so focused on one issue. Domestic violence, cancer, depression,

> financial strain, losing houses, relationship strain, despair, social disconnection, neglect of chronic health issues, loneliness, people dying alone, fear of contact with others in the context of COVID, children missing a year of school and socialisation, children living with hidden domestic violence, women living with hidden violence.
>
> *Senior doctor, emergency department, female, age 41–50*

> The risk of COVID is disproportionate to the current lockdown we are in. The economy, job losses, mental health issues, loneliness, and the inability to see family and friends has more of an impact than a virus that generally doesn't make us unwell.
>
> *Nurse, female, age 41–50*

A few argued that we need to learn to live with the virus.

> As time has gone on the pandemic has become challenging both professionally and personally. It may be better to take the Swedish approach and just let it run its course.
>
> *Nurse, hospital aged care, male, age 51–64*

> I have been nursing for over 30 years and worked in worse conditions in some countries overseas. … It is unrealistic and illogical to expect a germ-free society since our world began and we will never eradicate it either. So, the best way is just to continue giving care the best way we can by allowing people to make informed choices and live their lives as they see fit.
>
> *Nurse, emergency department, female, age 51–64*

> I think a lot of people have become unduly panic-stricken. To be honest the personal risks for most healthcare workers from COVID-19 are low. (I totally understand the concern about spreading to other family members and close contacts). Pandemics can get a lot worse than this. We signed up for healthcare and we have to be resilient—and most are of course. I don't think we should dial the panic meter up any higher than it already is. Maybe not a popular point of view right now, but you asked for my opinion and there it is!
>
> *Senior doctor, respiratory medicine, male, age 51–64*

As we discuss further in Chapter 13, healthcare workers were also worried about the impacts of lockdown on mental health and patient care.

> The lockdowns are extremely dangerous for some people's mental health as seen by my patients with increased alcohol abuse and drug use.
>
> *Podiatry, community care, female, age 20–30*

My personal experience has been that the lockdowns—and their consequences—have been worse for my mental health, and the mental health of my peers, than managing COVID in the hospital.

Junior doctor, hospital aged care, female, age 31–40

No matter how much support is out there, the virus is not going to disappear anytime soon. Having a closed society is probably as bad as the disease itself. People are going to die no matter what we do. I'm concerned about the number of deaths related to not accessing regular healthcare due to the pandemic.

Senior doctor, hospital aged care, male, age 51–64

The government's response is taking a huge toll on the population, one that is abnormal and devastating ... A more moderate and real approach would be far better for quality of life and healthy livelihoods. The states should all have the same rules ... The impact of the response is enormous.

Administrative worker, cardiology, female, age 41–50

The government is continuing to make its decisions based on the physical impact and number of deaths from COVID, over the short- and long-term effects on the population's mental health. Considering the length of time the pandemic has gone on, I feel the government is unrealistic in trying to maintain such harsh lockdown rules.

Nurse, infectious diseases, female, age 41–50

I am afraid that all the talk in the world will not right the mental health damage this pandemic, and the restrictions, has done to a large part of the population.

Junior doctor, emergency department, female, age 31–40

4

SELF-CARE STRUGGLES AND STRATEGIES

> I hate the five-kilometre radius limitation. The beach and the sea have been my solace since childhood, and I have effectively been cut off from this. Diving in the water has always given me the sense of washing all my problems away, it is where I go to think and heal myself after 20 years in critical care. Immersion in water hydrates my soul.
>
> *Nurse, intensive care, female age 51–64*

Increasing stress and demands in the clinical environment and at home meant that healthcare workers regularly sacrificed their own needs to provide care for patients, colleagues, and their families. Basic needs—from getting enough sleep to having access to water and nutritious food at work—were frequently compromised, as was healthcare workers' sense of safety and social connection. Though healthcare workers recognised the importance of taking care of themselves during the pandemic, they often lacked the time, energy, and resources to do so. Despite these challenges, healthcare workers drew on an array of self-care strategies to sustain their wellbeing.

Fatigue and disrupted sleep

Working long hours at an often-frenetic pace, disrupted sleep, and feeling run-down with no time for recovery, were defining features of healthcare workers' experiences.

> I couldn't sleep, I was having night sweats, grinding my teeth, anxiety out of control. My desire to quit is higher than ever before.
>
> *Pharmacist, community care, female, age 41–50*

DOI: 10.4324/9781003228394-4

> There are times I feel claustrophobic at night because I can't go for a walk if I can't sleep. I feel isolated. I can't go to my usual chemist or supermarket as they are seven kilometres away. These things all impact negatively and I don't know how this can be sustained without the community (me) falling apart.
>
> *Nurse, emergency department, female, age 51–64*

> I often dream that I have mild symptoms, and experience stress over whether I should be calling in sick to work, or whether I'm leaving work short-staffed at the last minute, only to wake up and realise—again—that it was a dream.
>
> *Nurse, perioperative care, female, age 31–40*

Healthcare workers spoke about the negative effects of stress and fatigue on their physical health and their levels of concentration, motivation, and energy.

> I have struggled to sleep and concentrate every day for over five months (today is 28 August 2020).
>
> *Respiratory scientist, female, age 31–40*

> The fatigue of being on high alert is really starting to affect my concentration levels and my sleep. I'm finding it increasingly difficult to be optimistic or positive.
>
> *Nurse, medical specialty, female, age 20–30*

> I really find it hard to focus and concentrate which is quite new to me.
>
> *Physiotherapist, general medicine, female, age 41–50*

> I feel that COVID has not only had an impact emotionally, but that it manifests in the physical. I have developed cold sores and my skin has broken out during COVID. These are generally indicators to me—especially the cold sores—that my body is run down. I am tired and fatigued.
>
> *Nurse, palliative care, female, age 31–40*

> My main problems are a feeling of burnout, worsening health due to exhaustion, and too much alcohol.
>
> *Senior doctor, emergency department, female, age 51–64*

Some healthcare workers found it more difficult than usual to nurture their bodies with nutritious and enjoyable meals.

> I don't want to leave my home. I'd rather eat baked beans on toast than go to the supermarket on my own wearing a mask.
>
> *Nurse, COVID ward, female, age 51–64*

> I have no motivation to exercise or cook nutritious meals. I'm experiencing a higher than usual sense of self-loathing over my weight and concern over how I will manage it.
>
> *Nurse, perioperative care, female, age 31–40*

> I've gained three kilograms since the start of COVID and I am now doing zero exercise. I have lost my drive and excitement for going outside and doing things outside the home.
>
> *Clinical scientist, medical specialty, female, age 41–50*

> Doing shift work made it hard to get to the shops and when I did, I couldn't even get my essential items like frozen vegetables or meat. So, I lived off yoghurt for two months. Designated shopping hours for healthcare workers, outside of the usual 9am to 5pm would help.
>
> *Nurse, emergency department, female, age 20–30*

Rest and recovery

Increased work and family obligations and stresses left many healthcare workers reporting that they had limited opportunities for respite and recovery at work and at home.

> There is no reprieve. Most people are stressed about staying home and being isolated, but working on the frontline is another dimension. We need some reprieve.
>
> *Senior doctor, emergency department, female, age 41–50*

> It would be nice to have more days off. I would be happy to work longer days to have a longer weekend to spend time with my family and cats. I would feel more well-rested this way. Weekends are too short when you have family obligations, and you end up feeling just as fatigued with less time to rest.
>
> *Pharmacist, hospital, female, age 20–30*

> In healthcare, there's no space or flexibility for an "off" moment or day. You have to give 100 percent of your energy, all day, every day. It's really difficult when you're already stressed and fatigued. Week-on week-off rostering systems during times like this should be considered to maintain a sustainable workforce.
>
> *Speech pathologist, rehabilitation, female, age 31–40*

> Rostering needs to be improved so that workers can plan activities that support their wellbeing. The current roster I work under comes out with less than a week's notice and it means I cannot look after myself or family properly.
>
> *Medical scientist, infectious diseases, female, age 31–40*

Finding time and energy for self-care amidst all the other demands of the pandemic was challenging. For some, caring for themselves felt like one more thing to do on an already overburdened to-do list.

> I definitely feel the lockdown is making it harder to access help, due to ongoing responsibilities with my kids and not being able to physically see a doctor.
>
> *Nurse, intensive care, female, age 31–40*

> I have not been taking care of myself at all. I've been too busy and stressed looking after my patients, staff and business.
>
> *General practitioner, female, age 41–50*

> I feel really withdrawn. I know there are lots of supports available but I don't want to reach out. I just want to hide until it's all over but, somehow, we have to keep going every day. Quitting social media has been the best thing for me—I was feeling triggered by selfish people undermining the tireless commitment of health care workers.
>
> *Physiotherapist, community care, female, age 31–40*

> There is a big divide between telling people to "take time out to refresh" and the realities of being able to take time out of work. In this pandemic there has never been a "good" time to be able to walk away and refresh. It is constant as the work needs to be done. I have found that when I get home, I am exhausted.
>
> *Nurse, emergency department, female, age 51–64*

Healthcare workers also expressed a reluctance to take holiday leave during lockdown, as there was nowhere to go, and they wanted to save their leave to be able to see their families.

> It's hard for me to justify taking annual leave, as it seems like a waste.
>
> *Physiotherapist, intensive care, female, age 31–40*

> Burning through annual leave concerns me, as when the time comes that we can see our friends, I want to be able to spend that little extra time with interstate family, or take a few extra days camping to make up for a year of waking up, coming to work then going to sleep, all to repeat it the next day.
>
> *Administrative worker, radiology, female, age 20–30*

Struggling to self-care

Due to lockdown restrictions and increasing workplace demands, healthcare workers described losing many of their usual strategies for coping with stress and anxiety, such as spending time with friends and family, going to the gym, or visiting places of sanctuary. Some struggled to find alternative ways to take care of themselves.

Normally I would be able to fill my bucket which enabled me to cope with the challenges of working in health care. My weekends would involve seeing friends, laughing, smiling, dancing. I would spend time with my family and niece and nephews. Due to isolation, I have not been able to do these things so my ability to cope with challenges of work has been much less, my resilience a lot lower.

Occupational therapist, palliative care, female, age 20–30

My best coping mechanism was training in martial arts. That has been taken away. If you continually strip coping mechanisms from people, are you really surprised that people are struggling to deal with the world?

Technician, emergency department, male, age 41–50

In a job that is stressful at the best of times, I have found it the hardest to not be able to utilise my usual coping mechanisms: socialising, seeing my family in New Zealand, or leaving my house or area on my days off.

Nurse, intensive care, female, age 20–30

I struggle with the feeling of being imprisoned in my own home, not being able to engage with my family and friends as I want and need. My work is draining and demanding but at the same time enjoyable. Not being able to enjoy my home life is not good for my mental well-being. I have worked hard to reach a "happy medium". This current situation has decimated this concept for me.

Dentist, emergency department, female, age 51–64

I'm a person who maintains my high level of well-being by using successful coping mechanisms such as exercising at the gym, spending time with friends and family and treating myself to a self-care day (hair, nails, shopping etc.). My whole routine has been thrown off and I can't do any of the things I used to do to cope.

Administrative worker, medical specialty, female, age 20–30

Normal emotional supports such as visiting with family and friends, group sport, and simple things like hugs were gone during the early stages of restrictions.

Occupational therapist, community care, female, age 51–64

The impact of not being able to go to the gym—for those that regularly do—has been enormous. I have gotten to a point where I am agitated, restless, and less like myself as I don't have the same outlet I used to. Although we can exercise at home, and outside for limited times, it is nowhere near the same and should be recognised as essential.

Occupational therapist, medical specialty, female, age 20–30

> Anyone who can't self-sedate with Netflix and junk food is having their life completely destroyed by lockdown.
>
> *Junior doctor, intensive care, male, age 31–40*

Self-care strategies that worked

Despite these challenges, many healthcare workers identified coping strategies that they found helpful to sustain their own wellbeing while continuing to care for others during the pandemic.

> Keeping it simple, refocusing on self-care as the utmost priority has helped.
>
> *Nurse, mental health, female, age 41–50*

Some were able to draw on existing coping strategies to help them during the crisis.

> The best supports are those already established. I am finding I have no mental space for new information, so I am relying heavily on my known relaxation activities.
>
> *Senior doctor, anaesthetics, female, age 31–40*

> Many years ago I did a mindfulness-based stress reduction course. I have drawn on this in the past and believe it has helped me again through COVID. Psychoeducation, and understanding why things are happening and what you can do to influence how you experience them, is highly important and should be learning available to all frontline healthcare workers. Emergency services do this a bit. Psychologists integrate it into their practice. Most other health workers do not have any structured access to this opportunity.
>
> *General practitioner, female, age 31–40*

Others needed to be inventive in finding new ways of taking care of themselves. The quotes below show the spectrum of self-care activities that healthcare workers employed to "stay afloat" during the pandemic.

Arts and leisure

Some healthcare workers told us about finding joy in the arts—novels, films, music, journaling, and even "mindless" television—to distract from the darkness at work.

> The arts are absolutely vital. Singing and dancing to a favourite song, gazing at a favourite painting, reading a great novel, or watching a beautifully made film—these have lifted my spirits time and again.
>
> *General practitioner, female, age 31–40*

> Watching mindless television shows.
>
> *Senior doctor, medical specialty, female, age 51–64*

Playing a guitar. Writing a diary.

Nurse, radiology, female, age 51–64

I'm doing a journal which has helped me. I have focussed on that rather than getting depressed with the news in the papers and on the television. I have included articles in my journal, and personal little bits of family information and have taken a lot of photos, mainly photos of signs which show compassion and caring.

Pharmacist, community care, female, age 51–64

Taking a break from anything medical. I am reading novels and watching documentaries about interesting people in my downtime.

General practitioner, female, age 51–64

Humour has been good for me. Watching funny YouTube videos about COVID and other humorous TV shows or stand-up gigs on Netflix. Also playing trivia games has been fun and watching TV with nothing to do with COVID-19 has been a good escape.

Allied health practitioner, medical specialty, female, age 41–50

Physical exercise and nutrition

With gyms and exercise studios closed due to the lockdown, many healthcare workers turned to new forms of exercise that could be done within the confines of their home, or within their one-hour window of outdoor exercise in their five-kilometre zone. Walking, running, cycling, and yoga were among the most popular.

Being allowed to exercise with others has been helpful to help maintain my sanity and connection with friends during these times.

Nurse, intensive care, female, age 41–50

Yoga via YouTube and the Down Dog yoga app, walking with a friend, have all been amazing.

Occupational therapist, emergency department, female, age 31–40

Distracting myself at home really helps. Having a goal to run five kilometres without stopping.

Nurse, emergency department, female, age 20–30

I'm quite enjoying lockdown as I can cycle on the roads, and I am enjoying exploring every part of my five-kilometre radius.

General practitioner, female, age 65–70

> I've been dancing at home to online dance classes which has been great for my physical and mental health.
>
> *Nurse, palliative care, female, age 31–40*

Several healthcare workers told us that they had reduced their alcohol intake as part of their self-care, while others looked forward to a drink at the end of a stressful work day.

> I've deliberately stopped drinking alcohol during the pandemic. Previously I would have one to two glasses of wine per week but I lost my appetite for it when I was stressed about COVID in March, and could see how easy it would be to increase intake. Lack of alcohol and riding my bike 17 kilometres each way to work has been invaluable in keeping me afloat during this time.
>
> *Senior doctor, general medicine, female, age 41–50*

> One of the big things for me was stopping my alcohol intake. At the start of the pandemic my alcohol intake definitely increased and obviously that makes you feel worse. I then did dry July during a time when I previously would've felt I "most needed" alcohol and this helped me enormously. I felt physically a lot better and mentally too.
>
> *Nurse, general medicine, female, age 20–30*

> What has helped? Gin!
>
> *General practitioner, female, age 51–64*

Like many other Australians, some healthcare workers took up bread making as a relaxing activity that made the most of long days at home.

> I forgot to mention how much pleasure I got from cooking and making sourdough bread. A rather trivial but wonderful strategy my whole family benefited from.
>
> *Senior doctor, medical specialty, female, age 41–50*

Animals and nature

Animals provided companionship and joy, especially for those living alone.

> Everyone should have a pet!
>
> *General practitioner, female, age 31–40*

> Patting my cat, following animal stories on Facebook.
>
> *Nurse, community care, female, age 51–64*

> Walking in nature with my dog and having friends to walk and talk with has saved me.
>
> *Senior doctor, surgical, female, age 41–50*

Natural green spaces offered a source of solace.

> I try to just appreciate the little things, like blossoms on trees or the call of a magpie for a moment of grounding.
>
> *Administrative worker, surgical, female, age 31–40*

> Spending more time outdoors with quiet time has been helpful for me.
>
> *Senior doctor, manager, female, age 51–64*

> Getting outdoors in natural beauty has been amazing for my mental health. I cannot recommend the preservation of our green spaces more. They are critical for us to move forward in a positive way.
>
> *Senior doctor, medical specialty, female, age 31–40*

Routines and boundaries

Maintaining routines, and establishing boundaries around work, created a sense of structure for some healthcare workers.

> I continued with usual daily activities as much as possible and maintained a focus on family. I stopped listening to the media and this made a huge impact.
>
> *Social worker, hospital aged care, female, age 41–50*

> My partner and I planned every day, including exercise and coffee time, and had a great time catching up on things around the house, gardening, cleaning out cupboards etc.
>
> *Paramedic, male, age 51–64*

> Setting limits and boundaries for myself … aiming to leave work on time is ongoing.
>
> *Occupational therapist, general medicine, female, age 41–50*

> I try to get up daily early, even if I am not working, shower, dress well, makeup, exercise. I am trying to focus on what I am going to do after lockdown. I have recognised that I suffer stress more when we are not locked down by the daily grind of life, and COVID has been a peaceful time for reflection of what is important in life.
>
> *Nurse, emergency department, female, age 41–50*

> Certainly, having a few small positive things to focus on each week is very helpful in getting through this—no different to the strategies we generally employ with clients who experience these sorts of feelings.
>
> *Social worker, community care, female, age 51–64*

Hope, faith, and spirituality

Some healthcare workers discussed the importance of faith or spirituality and the value of staying connected with their faith community.

> I have a faith. That makes a difference for me.
>
> *Nurse, emergency department, female, age 41–50*

> I feel incredibly privileged to have employment through the pandemic. I have been well supported by my faith community which includes many other health care workers; and I feel incredibly thankful for a fairly grounded sense of resilience.
>
> *Nurse, palliative care, female, age 51–64*

> Reading spiritual philosophy.
>
> *Nurse, community care, female, age 51–64*

> Reading more on Buddhism helped me to view the pandemic in less of a negative light, and more as a life challenge. What can we learn about ourselves and others?
>
> *Nurse, emergency department, female, age 20–30*

> My faith is central to how I cope.
>
> *Psychologist, private practice, female, age 41–50*

Others spoke about the importance of maintaining hope and making future plans during the pandemic.

> I'm looking forward to being able to go to the beach and spend more time with my family.
>
> *Senior doctor, infectious diseases, male, age 41–50*

> I'm really looking forward to seeing my family and praying that we have a happy Christmas.
>
> *Nurse, surgical, female, age 20–30*

> A vaccine would be nice!
>
> *Pharmacist, emergency department, male, age 31-40*

> This will be over soon, and we will have normal life again. I am very hopeful.
>
> *Administrative worker, infectious diseases, female, age 31–40*

Mindfulness and relaxation helped with staying in the present.

> I read a phrase on Instagram: "The little boy said to the horse 'I cannot see ahead, it is too foggy' and the horse said to the little boy 'can you see your feet?' The little boy said 'yes' and the horse said 'then just take one step'." I try to remember this to bring my mind back to the present.
>
> *Nurse, respiratory medicine, female, age 65–70*

> Some years ago, I did a mindfulness for stress relief course. I learned so much about dealing with workplace stress, how to put things in perspective, how to ask for support and how to give it, great meditation techniques. Best thing I've ever done. Mindfulness meditation has helped me a lot in dealing with stress.
>
> *Nurse, hospital-based, female, age 51–64*

> Weekly evening sessions of mindfulness meditation done as a group online with a very good facilitator made a lot of difference. I feel calmer and more balanced.
>
> *Administrative worker, non-clinical, female, age 51–64*

> Meditation and yogic breathing exercises have been the most helpful.
>
> *Senior doctor, intensive care, female, age 41–50*

Healthcare workers told us about smartphone apps they had found useful for mindfulness and relaxation.

> The Youper [mental health] app saved my sanity, getting me to check-in daily and doing mindfulness exercises. I didn't want to do them but did them anyway because I had hit rock bottom emotionally.
>
> *Nurse, respiratory medicine, female, age 51–64*

> Mindfulness techniques on Calm have helped me a lot. Online supports about how to deal with COVID and work in healthcare have been great.
>
> *Allied health practitioner, medical specialty, female, age 41–50*

> As a team, we have been using the Smiling Mind [meditation] app at work after a shift, I find this is a great way to end the shift, and a great team building exercise.
>
> *Nurse, palliative care, female, age 20–30*

> I already had some well-being strategies in place. Since COVID I have been using the HeadSpace app several times a week. If I can't sleep or am feeling anxious, I put it on.
>
> *Senior doctor, anaesthetics, female, age 41–50*

> This Way Up [cognitive behavioural therapy program] is great. Doctors need insight into their own mental health before they can help others.
>
> *General practitioner, female, age 51–64*

For some healthcare workers, alternative remedies were helpful.

> I extensively use the support of universal medicine practitioners and therapies, as they help me to reconnect back to that still place within, the essence of my soul, and to come back from being drawn into the drama.
>
> *Junior doctor, general medicine, female, age 31–40*

> Being self-aware and self-monitoring. I have also taught myself some basic reflexology.
>
> *Nurse, community care, female, age 51–64*

Self-acceptance and self-compassion

Some healthcare workers talked about the importance of accepting things as they are.

> I generally feel good about the things I can control, and I try not to dwell on the things I can't control.
>
> *Nurse, emergency department, female, age 51–64*

> There are lots of things causing stress that can't be controlled. Therefore, I think the main option for me is to acknowledge the stress and anxiety, and that it is there for a good reason, and to give myself permission to feel it. Then I can get on with the things I need to get done.
>
> *Junior doctor, anaesthetics, female, age 31–40*

> This experience has refocussed my resolve to concentrate on the important things, and to advocate for the vulnerable at every opportunity. I now have a simple philosophy: 1) be a good person, 2) have a lot of fun, 3) give few fucks about things you can't change.
>
> *Senior doctor, residential aged care, male, age 31–40*

Healthcare workers also wrote about the value of being kind and forgiving towards themselves and others during these difficult times.

> Self-care, and trying to enjoy family time, without thinking about all the chores that have to be done due to working so much more than usual.
>
> *Nurse, perioperative care, female, age 20–30*

> Reminders to be kind and gentle to myself have been positive.
>
> *Nurse, palliative care, female, age 51–64*

> Being kind and compassionate to myself and allowing myself to take it easier than I would normally. Engaging in activities that allow me self-care and increase my exercise and general wellbeing.
>
> *Psychologist, medical specialty, female, age 20–30*

> Although I have experienced some symptoms of anxiety and depression, this is not something I am concerned about as I feel this is quite normal for the times.
>
> *Physiotherapist, respiratory medicine, female, age 20–30*

> I'm wondering whether there's no way to really avoid feeling bad during this time and it may be a case of just learning how to deal with that and knowing that afterwards there may have to be some intensive work to get back to balance.
>
> *Senior doctor, infectious diseases, female, age 41–50*

Acknowledgement of vulnerability, as an integral part of being human, was also described.

> We all want the best for colleagues, clients, our managers, the organisation, but we're human; there should not be so much tacit pressure on staff to just handle anything that's imposed without any consultation. Of course, in the midst of the urgent necessary planning for healthcare to cope with the pandemic, it has been appropriate for assertive decision-making and for staff to accept orders, but that shouldn't become habitual and extend to everything. So mostly I'm saying there's not enough plain talk about human frailty and the limitations of lifestyle strategies and apps (not that I am totally discounting these either). Sometimes I'm just going to fall apart and that's normal in this abnormal situation—as much for me as any other human (client or staff).
>
> *Allied health practitioner, community care, female, age 65–70*

5

THE IMPOSSIBLE JUGGLE OF WORK AND CARE

> It has been the hardest part of my life to juggle work, home schooling, study, and working from home. There is not enough quiet space to work at home and we all need some time apart. I feel like I haven't done anything well.
>
> *Nurse, medical specialty, female, age 31–40*

Working from home became the "new normal" for many Australians during the pandemic. But this was not an option for many delivering frontline healthcare. Our survey found that more than a quarter of healthcare workers had primary caring responsibilities at home. Almost as many had children who were home-schooling. Healthcare workers working from home juggled these responsibilities with the provision of patient care. School and childcare became more difficult to access for many, even though there were government provisions for "essential workers". The juggle of work and care was even harder for those who had caring responsibilities for both children and older relatives, the so-called "sandwich generation". Healthcare workers worried a lot about how the pandemic impacted their families. Not surprisingly, the healthcare workers in our study most likely to report caring responsibilities were women aged between 31 and 50 years. Many shared their views about gender disparities in the workplace and the consequences of increased carer responsibilities for their careers.

The "insane" juggle of increased home and work demands

In writing about their experiences, healthcare workers provided an account of the impossibility of juggling work, which had become more demanding, and care (including home-schooling), which had also become extremely stressful. This was accompanied by feelings of guilt and being judged by others. The feeling that "I'm not doing anything well" was evident throughout their responses.

DOI: 10.4324/9781003228394-5

For the healthcare workers who are juggling care it's insane.

Psychologist, community care, female, age 31–40

We have been expected to still show up for our jobs, with further stress and worry, and then also go home and home-school and care for our children and attend to all home duties as well. It's been difficult to have flexibility at work and with home-schooling to come to a reasonable balance between everything. We have been denied time off work to assist at home, and then are shamed for "allowing our children to fall behind".

Nurse, emergency department, female, age 20–30

Being in a two-doctor household—both with patient-facing roles—while having an academic role, whilst also home-schooling has been nearly impossible.

Senior doctor, anaesthetics, female, age 41–50

Increased work hours plus home-schooling children is impossible: both are a high priority.

Nurse, community care, female, age 41–50

Remote [home-school] learning has been one of the hardest challenges during this pandemic.

Nurse, medical specialty, female, age 41–50

I worry a lot about the practical aspects of caring for my children whilst continuing to try and work.

Senior doctor, anaesthetics, male, age 31–40

It's hard home-schooling and working. I feel like I let my children down. At one point my husband couldn't work from home, so I had to use annual leave to school my children. It caused a lot of stress and I felt like I was letting my workplace down. Couldn't win! My children are looking after themselves.

Nurse, emergency department, female, age 41–50

I'm a supervisor for junior doctors, so helping them through this difficult period, on top of work and home-schooling young children, has been particularly hard.

Senior doctor, emergency department, female, age 31–40

I took time off private work for some weeks for home-schooling.

Senior doctor, anaesthetics, female, age 41–50

> The main challenge has been the guilt of seeing everybody else staying at home with kids, while I am leaving my 9-year-old with his 21-year-old university age brother.
>
> *Nurse, medical specialty, female, age 51–64*

Healthcare workers wrote about the exhaustion and the strain of additional caring responsibilities, along with the challenges of changing family dynamics.

> The strain of caring for elderly parents, or trying to keep them safe, while still having all of the work commitments and home life is the extra strain that I have noticed during the pandemic.
>
> *Nurse, emergency department, female, age 51–64*

> I'm caring for an elderly parent and juggling working from home and supporting children with home-schooling. I often felt guilty that I did not redeploy to the front line.
>
> *Nurse, palliative care, female, age 51–64*

> Having a teenager with special needs remote learning whilst trying to work almost full time has been exhausting, but I felt I had to keep struggling along as the other two staff had younger kids with more issues. I carry guilt that my child and her needs get put after work priorities.
>
> *Administrative worker, surgical, female, age 31–40*

> Dealing with school and childcare has been extremely exhausting.
>
> *Senior doctor, medical specialty, female, age 41–50*

> Home-schooling on top of all this has been draining.
>
> *Administrative worker, general medicine, female, age 31–40*

> Restrictions on home and study have made this year harder than it would have been, which creates a lot of tension for family situations.
>
> *Administrative worker, hospital aged care, female, age 51–64*

> Like many people, I have been juggling with very complex family dynamics. Managing work from home and staying at home to comply with isolation rules in my workplace, has really put a strain on me.
>
> *Social worker, medical specialty, female, age 51–64*

> I have four kids at three different schools and I get emails about webinars for resilience or wellbeing from each of the schools, multiple times per week. It is absolutely exhausting having to keep up with personal and work emails.
>
> *Nurse, community care, female, age 31–40*

Sole parents

Sole parents wrote about the distinct challenges of their caring responsibilities; and the additional struggles that they experienced as they tried to manage both care and work responsibilities without their usual supports.

> Mostly I feel I have let my sons down. They are home-schooling, yet I am never home as a single parent. I work three jobs for three different sites which has a big impact on healthcare workers. I would gladly work for one employer if I could, but the three jobs allowed me to spend time with my sons when they went to school drop-off and pick-ups. Now, when they have needed me home, I can't be as my jobs can't be done remotely. I give everything to my jobs, yet my sons get very little of me. When I'm home I'm generally exhausted.
>
> *Nurse, intensive care, female, age 41–50*

> Being a single mother, working full-time and home-schooling three children full time, has been a huge stress on top of COVID stress. There is no reprieve.
>
> *Senior doctor, emergency department, female, age 41–50*

> It is difficult being a single mother of two small boys, one doing remote learning in Prep [first year of primary school] several days per week, the other with developmental delays (accessing allied health support via Zoom) with being a healthcare worker.
>
> *Senior doctor, medical specialty, female, age 41–50*

> My work is more stressful and hard—I work in cancer care and we are keeping a BUNCH of patients out of hospital due to visitor restrictions and fears. Added to this: intermittent failure of delivery shopping, no cleaner, and the fucking home schooling. I am a single parent of three kids and the youngest is really incapable of organising herself to do schoolwork while I am at work.
>
> *Senior doctor, medical specialty, female, age 41–50*

Worries about children and older family members

Throughout their accounts, healthcare workers told us of their worries about those close to them, especially their children and elderly parents.

Healthcare workers shared their concerns about the burden of the pandemic on their children.

> The main challenge is the wellbeing of the families of healthcare workers, especially the children. Already during this time, the mental health of our children is greatly impacted. For children of healthcare workers there is the

> added stressor of knowing that mum or dad are dealing directly with COVID patients, increasing their worry for their parent, as well as their own safety concerns. Media exposure—which is difficult to avoid—is also a concern for our children as healthcare worker infections are reported. Increased hours away from the family. Some older children were home alone, with both parents working as essential workers. These kids not only navigate online schooling alone, but have the concerns as mentioned above regarding their healthcare worker parents.
>
> *Nurse, intensive care, female, age 51–64*

> I'm struggling to help with my children's sense of sadness and hopelessness due to the pandemic.
>
> *Senior doctor, medical specialty, female, age 51–64*

These worries traversed all aspects of their children's lives during the pandemic, all ages, and all life stages.

> I had to stop breastfeeding my baby, as my workplace told me that they couldn't afford for me to have a pumping break. I was not at all ready for him to be weaned.
>
> *Nurse, surgical, female, age 31–40*

> My three-year-old son has autism spectrum disorder and is a very poor sleeper.
>
> *Nurse, emergency department, male, age 41–50*

> Changes to childcare brought behaviour disturbance, adding to my exhaustion.
>
> *Physiotherapist, community care, female, age 31–40*

> My son's visits to me were stopped by his mother solely due to me working in the high-risk areas of health.
>
> *Nurse, intensive care, male, age 51–64*

> My children are disadvantaged while I have to work extra unpaid hours to provide healthcare. I am not home enough and am too exhausted to be an effective, caring parent.
>
> *Nurse, community care, male, age 41–50*

> My kids can't do swimming lessons, socialising, identify facial expressions due to masks etc.
>
> *General practitioner, male, age 31–40*

> School time lost. Too much sitting and screen time. Lack of exercise.
>
> *Senior doctor, medical specialty, female, age 41–50*

> Their sporting careers, their education, and their social skills.
>
> *Physiotherapist, community care, male, age 51–64*

> The stress of having to have a plan for your family if you do get COVID or even die from it. Watching the kids stressed every time I leave for work and they can't touch me until I shower when I get home.
>
> *Nurse, emergency department, female, age 41–50*

> My daughter has had her Year 12 [final school year] pretty much ruined by this. I am very, very sad for her.
>
> *Senior doctor, emergency department, male, age 51–64*

> My daughter is a graduate nurse, who was exposed to a COVID patient without full PPE. I felt awful as she was in Melbourne—and I am regional—so I could not care for her if she got sick.
>
> *Nurse, community care, female, age 41–50*

> My three young adult children at home are unable to see their friends, go to university or do "normal" things. I worry for them.
>
> *Nurse, palliative care, female, age 51–64*

Whether providing primary care, or supporting them in other ways, healthcare workers struggled with concerns about their elderly relatives as restrictions reduced opportunities for contact.

> The hardest challenge has been thinking about who would look after my father if I got ill.
>
> *Senior doctor, anaesthetics, female, age 41–50*

> It has had a huge impact on elderly parents, especially those in aged care and this is an added worry for me; not able to take time off to care for my elderly mother because I would feel guilty about being away from work.
>
> *Physiotherapist, respiratory medicine, female, age 65–70*

> I'm more worried about being a carer for my elderly mother than anything else. I do not want to accidentally pass on the virus to my family, especially mum.
>
> *Nurse, emergency department, female, age 51–64*

> I have been responsible for providing support for my mother—who lives alone—and for my husband, both of whom suffer from depression and anxiety, made worse by the pandemic.
>
> *Clinical scientist, pathology, female, age 51–64*

> It has been hard dealing with my mother's medical appointments and mental health issues involving her comorbidities. All the while still trying to keep her positive and working long hours trying to keep up with my work demands. It's been exhausting mentally, emotionally and physically. I shouldn't complain. At least my workplace was flexible with my hours to enable me to coordinate my mother's medical situation, but not having other family to help has been tough.
>
> *Administrative worker, surgical, female, age 51–64*

> I believe that COVID restrictions on my family have more of a negative impact on my mental health than my COVID work; for example, not being able to visit my 97-year-old father or see and care for my grandchildren!
>
> *Administrative worker, community care, female, age 65–70*

> I am very concerned about my 80-year-old mother living alone, I haven't been able to see her.
>
> *Nurse, surgical, female, age 51–64*

> My stressors are not being able to see my mother in her aged care facility and ensuring my father, who lives alone and is independent, is OK.
>
> *Nurse, community care, female, age 41–50*

> My father, who was an aged care resident, contracted COVID-19 and was hospitalised for five weeks. This stress of not being able to see him, on top of working in the healthcare system, has been a lot to deal with.
>
> *Nurse, medical specialty, female, age 31–40*

Spillover

For many healthcare workers, the boundaries between home and work blurred as work increasingly spilled over into their home environment. This was not only the case for those working from home. Even for those still providing face-to-face care, leaving the workplace did not necessarily mean leaving work responsibilities behind. This spillover from work to home generated feelings of guilt about what healthcare workers "should" be doing; and the tensions in trying to meet the competing demands.

> On my days off, I should be looking after my four- and ten-year-old daughters. But I am so distracted by emails, phone calls from distressed staff, extra work, trying to obtain masks, Zoom meetings etc that my children have suffered.
>
> *Senior doctor, anaesthetics, female, age 41–50*

> Staff were forced to use their personal phone for Zoom, telehealth, and phone calls, when they were required to work from home. Making it difficult at times to switch-off from work.
>
> *Speech pathologist, community care, female, age 51–64*

> I would like to manage my workload so I can switch off when home, and care for my children.
>
> *Nurse, aged care, female, age 41–50*

> The main challenge has been being unable to have work-life balance during Stage Four lockdown. I have appreciated having a stable job but have not really been able to switch off easily.
>
> *Physiotherapist, intensive care, male, age 31–40*

> Many days I have felt exhausted and frustrated because I've done a lot, but nothing very well.
>
> *Administrative worker, palliative care, female, age 41–50*

No space for me

Many healthcare workers with children struggled with the competing demands of being a responsible worker and a good parent. Their attempts to meet the needs of those around them often came at the expense of their own needs.

> My main issue is I need some time ON MY OWN!! But working part time, and with three children under five to home-school and care for, I feel I am unable to EVER get quiet alone time.
>
> *Radiographer, emergency department, female, age 31–40*

> I have struggled with being an employee and a mother of three children all at school. I can't seem to fit all the demands on me into a day well—so I found self-care was the first thing to go, which didn't help me sustain my strength for the situation.
>
> *Administrative worker, palliative care, female, age 41–50*

> I am hammered all day at work, then come home to the household that is working and schooling from home. They "want to talk" when all I want to do is sit quietly.
>
> *Nurse, medical specialty, female, age 51–64*

> Even using all supports around us, the strain on wellbeing is profound. The hardest part is the lack of ability to take a proper break. If not working, then home-schooling or parenting. The ability to recharge is not present.
>
> *Occupational therapist, community care, female, age 31–40*

> The loss of routine, with no "me time", was the most stressful. Trying to keep home-schooling momentum going, then having to go to work and being

in-charge and "on" ... when all I wanted to do was cry in the corner because some days had been spent with three hours of yelling and trying to keep everyone from having a meltdown.

Nurse, intensive care, female, age 41–50

It was very isolating being at home trying to teach remotely and home-school my kids at the same time.

Junior doctor, emergency department, female, age 41–50

I think the combination of having to teach my children at home on my days off work and being made to feel bad for requiring onsite help at school when I did work, was what pushed me over the line. No downtime alone has been really hard coupled with significant limitations on how I can outwork my stress when I'm not at work.

Nurse, intensive care, female, age 41–50

Maintaining and supporting my children with school—one of them with special needs—and working leaves absolutely no time to manage anything stress-related. We need more acknowledgment and flexibility for workers with children who need to school from home.

Social worker, respiratory medicine, female, age 41–50

Home-schooling three primary-school aged children, and having a baby, and going back to help in the emergency department because of COVID-19. Right now, I'm not the priority.

Nurse, emergency department, female, age 31–40

It has been the hardest thing I have had to deal with in my nursing career, both for me and my family.

Nurse, emergency department, female, age 31–40

There's never been a more challenging time in my experience as a paediatrician. Managing patients, checking in on my staff's mental health, managing my family with my husband unemployed, and one son still in senior school. I feel I'm not looking out for me as there's nothing left in the tank!

Senior doctor, medical specialty, female, age 51–64

Working from home

Some healthcare workers wrote about the positive benefits of working from home, when possible.

> Working from home has had benefits. Productivity is improved as I am able to keep up with paperwork and documentation without distractions of others in the office.
>
> *Nurse, community care, female, age 41–50*

> Since the COVID-19 pandemic started, I have been working from home. I work three days per week. I have appreciated working from home as I had breast cancer last year and have co-morbidities.
>
> *Administrative worker, community care, female, age 51–64*

> Working from home two days a week, and two days a week in the office, has improved my physical, mental, and emotional health considerably!
>
> *Administrative worker, infectious diseases, female, age 51–64*

> Flexibility to work from home (including providing required equipment quickly) made the transition away from and back to the workplace relatively straightforward, which helped keep stress in check.
>
> *Psychologist, community care, female, age 51–64*

Gender, the life-course, and work

As they grappled with increased demands at home and at work, healthcare workers reflected on how their struggle exemplified gender inequalities at work and in society. They pointed out the imbalance in taking on additional caring responsibilities, described little understanding from male colleagues, and expressed concern about the future consequences for women's careers.

> It feels harder for us women who also take on so much of the schooling and domestic tasks as well.
>
> *Occupational therapist, medical specialty, female, age 41–50*

> Having a caring role for my young pre-school aged children, and also my elderly mother, is even more challenging during the pandemic. I feel that my (older, male) colleagues have little understanding of how challenging this is. The pandemic has amplified sexism in the workplace.
>
> *Senior doctor, intensive care, female, age 31–40*

> There is a pervading attitude that: (a) women will deal with all the child rearing aspects; and (b) this means they are now fairly useless from an employment perspective. This will hurt their careers in ways that they cannot recover from. This will end up as a self-fulfilling prophecy without better recognition of the impact of COVID-19 on health workers who are mothers, and policy and financial steps taken to change this. Otherwise, we will see worsening of

> the current economic and senior leadership inequality between women and men.
>
> *Senior doctor, medical specialty, female, age 41–50*

> The impact on my productivity, as a female academic clinician, has felt much more severe than what I observe from my male peers.
>
> *Senior doctor, anaesthetics, female, age 41–50*

> I'm worried about women's rights and the quest for equality going backwards.
>
> *Senior doctor, medical specialty, female, age 41–50*

The demands of work also disrupted important life events. Particularly poignant are the stories that female healthcare workers shared about having a baby during the pandemic.

> I had to return from maternity leave four months early due to staff shortages. I feel that I was robbed of this time with my baby.
>
> *Senior doctor, emergency department, female, age 31–40*

> I'm pregnant and feel the hospital has offered me no support in this regard particularly given we are in the midst of a health crisis. The general attitude is that you need to leave if you're not happy, rather than the workplace having a systemic look at alternative duties that may be available, and the unique challenges a pregnant woman may face during the middle of a pandemic.
>
> *Social worker, medical specialty, female, age 20–30*

> I went through pregnancy and delivery during lockdown. Lack of support is very stressful. My partner was only allowed to visit two hours a day while in hospital, friends can't visit. I know many trainees are in similar positions currently, or worrying about how they will look after small babies, or be able to safely return to work if there is still a COVID outbreak at the end of maternity leave.
>
> *Junior doctor, emergency department, female, age 31–40*

Organisational flexibility and support

Throughout healthcare workers' experiences of trying to juggle home and work were calls for flexibility and greater support at a range of levels—from more workplace flexibility to greater societal recognition—as well as acknowledgement of the impact on families of restrictions.

> I wanted to be there for my children during home-schooling, and during the second lockdown I completely dropped the ball. We aim to share household

duties 50/50, but me working full-time is taking its toll. I am aiming for 60 hours per fortnight, but because I am male that won't happen. I suggested reduced hours and split shifts and the response was: "I want you to work 8 hours".

Support staff, facilities and maintenance, male, age 41–50

I need greater support to manage my full-time workload, plus my full-time caring load for two primary school aged children, plus all the household chores that can no longer be outsourced either due to lockdown restrictions (cleaning etc).

Senior doctor, medical specialty, female, age 41–50

Not being able to see my parents has wider implications: no family support, no help with school holiday care, no "break" from parenting.

Senior doctor, palliative care, female, age 41–50

More understanding of trying to work and juggle three small children, especially one with special needs, and a husband who also has to work.

Nurse, medical specialty, female, age 31–40

I'd love to see more support, flexibility, and understanding for frontline workers who are parents. Schools continuing to offer supervision for children of essential workers saved us from reducing hours at work, and from significant household stress. I believe people in leadership roles don't see that the strain of shift work is magnified by home-schooling and self-isolation. For many of them, their Monday to Friday lives haven't really changed much—for shift workers it's much worse. All the usual stresses plus PPE, angry relatives, kids at home and pissed-off partners because shifts start earlier and end later.

Nurse, intensive care, female, age 51–64

Working shift work, in particular night duty, it's very easy to burn out when caring for young children, remote teaching, then heading off to work night shift. Being awake for 24 hours continuously, and making critical decisions about patient care, isn't ideal. Subsidised accommodation or sleeping quarters or coordinated child-minding programs for shift workers with children would be well-received if this was ever to happen again.

Nurse, medical specialty, female, age 31–40

I think expectations around maintaining normal work output, despite not being able to access usual supports, has been a big part of burnout for me. The expectation to look after kids while working is unrealistic and exceptionally stressful. Working from home is very difficult when children are at home. It would be nice to see workplaces being understanding of the situation being challenging for parents, and relaxing expectations or increasing flexibility.

Senior doctor, medical specialty, female, age 31–40

6

MISSING THE HUMAN CONNECTION

> I think everyone has a degree of sadness about what we've lost.
>
> *Senior doctor, emergency department, female, age 41–50*

The pandemic disrupted usual ways of seeing family, friends, and familiar faces. While stay-at-home mandates and social distancing rules undoubtedly saved lives, they also contributed to what has been described as a "pandemic of loneliness". We begin this chapter with healthcare workers' accounts of the loss of anticipated rituals, events and celebrations. We then share their experiences of mourning the loss of everyday social relationships and connections: from young singles unable to meet a new partner, to grandparents missing the first year of a grandbaby's life. Many wrote about the inability to comfort loved ones or to grieve properly following the death of family or friends. Others described the challenges of maintaining relationships, particularly for those living alone or separated from their loved ones in another state or country. We conclude this chapter with words of advice from healthcare workers about the importance of staying connected with family and friends.

Loss of celebration and ritual

As for many people in the community, the impact of the pandemic and the resulting lockdown was felt in terms of loss—in particular, anticipated celebrations, rituals, and milestones that were unable to occur. Healthcare workers also wrote about "putting their life on hold" as planned events had to be cancelled.

> Grieving the loss of expected joys in 2020. I had to cancel my first holiday planned in years, can't see my nephews, no celebrations with family.
>
> *Nurse, emergency department, female, age 20–30*

DOI: 10.4324/9781003228394-6

Cancellation of all milestones associated with finishing medical school—graduation celebrations, dinners. Cancellation of plans over summer. I have spent seven years at university, and have never travelled, and now I don't know that I'll get the opportunity. Feeling like there is nothing to look forward to.

Student, female, age 20–30

Distance from family and friends, and the grief of lost or delayed potentials: not able to explore after moving to Melbourne, not having a partner.

Junior doctor, emergency department, female, age 31–40

Increasing loneliness, especially living alone and missing out on life milestones.

Pharmacist, community care, female, age 31–40

You feel like you are not doing either (home-school or work) as well as you normally would and guilty about the amount of screen-time your children have with little to do in Stage Four restrictions. Seven months of the same Groundhog Day with no holidays or proper breaks, constant caring, and keeping everyone else motivated to learn at work and at home. No life events to look forward to or milestones; joyful things have lessened.

Pharmacist, education, female, age 31–40

I am lucky to have my health and a loving family. However, I had a lot of plans this year and I have had to cancel all of them.

Nurse, medical specialty, female, age 20–30

Personal life being put on hold at my age; including not being able to go out and meet new people, with the view to meet a long-term partner and hopefully have a family down the track.

Speech pathologist, general medicine, female, age 31–40

Increased pressures at home with three young adult children and helping them adjust to lockdown and the grief of a year that has been lost to them.

Nurse, community care, female, age 51–64

Contracting COVID-19 and having to isolate. I found home isolation for two weeks quite challenging. It has also caused my partner and I to cancel our wedding this year which has been stressful.

Junior doctor, emergency department, male, age 20–30

People should know it is okay to mourn the loss of a planned trip, wedding, big party etc and not feel bad to say it. A lot of people are upset at the loss of these things but don't want to voice it as they feel there are bigger things happening.

Radiographer, emergency department, female, age 41–50

Along with the loss of planned events, social interactions and freedoms previously taken for granted were missed.

> I miss not being able to interact with fellow colleagues in a relaxed manner at work—we are discouraged from congregating in tea rooms, touching, hugging etc. It makes for a long and bleak day.
>
> *Senior doctor, anaesthetics, female, age 31–40*

> Loss of freedom. Not able to interact with people. Not being able to use the gym, go to the beach, or leave to go on hikes or travel.
>
> *Administrative worker, radiology, female, age 20–30*

> Maintaining relationships has been difficult. Walking outdoors for exercise sucks with masks. I feel trapped and like I can't breathe. I sometimes feel hopeless that our government doesn't understand. I respect the severity of this virus, however I don't accept the restrictions as necessary. I want to feel independent again. I miss going out. I miss socialising. We need to see movement and a pathway to re-opening in Victoria. I feel like my heart is mourning the death of Victoria.
>
> *Physiotherapist, intensive care, female, age 20–30*

Separation from loved ones

Many healthcare workers told us that the enforced separation from loved ones was one of the most painful parts of the pandemic.

> It is the forced separation—not only for us, but for those we care for—that is emotionally straining. Knowing it's the right thing to do, doesn't mean it emotionally feels good.
>
> *Nurse, surgical, female, age 41–50*

> Not being able to see friends or family takes a toll.
>
> *Nurse, intensive care, female, age 20–30*

> I miss my friends. I miss my family. I hate not knowing when I will see them next. I miss the freedom to plan to cross the state border.
>
> *Medical scientist, respiratory medicine, female, age 31–40*

> The hardest thing, for a lot of aspects of life, is the loss of camaraderie and spontaneous interactions, though in some ways this has improved as people have settled and checked in more.
>
> *Physiotherapist, surgical, female, age 20–30*

> My family and friends are an integral part of my support system. Lately, I have not spent time with my friends due to restrictions brought about by COVID-19. I would have loved to go for coffee with friends like I used to.
>
> *Nurse, surgical, female, age 41–50*

People spoke about the basic human need for touch, social connection, and community.

> I miss the physical touch of extended family—my parents and kids—through hugs.
>
> *Nurse, medical specialty, female, age 41–50*

> People are being made to feel guilty about being lonely and desperate for some human contact. Being unable to cope, and needing human contact, is not being callous about the health impact on vulnerable people. It's a basic human necessity.
>
> *Junior doctor, emergency department, female, age 31–40*

> People need social interactions.
>
> *Administrative worker, community care, female, age 31–40*

> I think we have realised the importance of touch, and therefore of not having any.
>
> *Nurse, non-clinical, male, age 31–40*

> The isolated lifestyle is really bothering me. I am a hugger and miss the touch.
>
> *Nurse, palliative care, female, age 51–64*

> Loss of social connections is terrible.
>
> *Nurse, agency and community care, female, age 51–64*

Not seeing children, grandchildren, or elderly relatives

Like many others in the community, healthcare workers grieved lost time with children, grandchildren, and elderly relatives: time that they would never get back.

> The hardest part of the pandemic has been being separated from family and friends. That social contact is easily my biggest loss. I have really struggled with not being able to see my daughter and other relatives, one being a newborn.
>
> *Administrative worker, general medicine, female, age 51–64*

My family live in the country and the inability to visit and socialise has been hard, however I understand the reasons for this. Hopefully restrictions will wind back soon and we can return to a "COVID-normal".

Nurse, palliative care, male, age 51–64

Not seeing my grandchildren and family has been very hard. Since March this year I feel as though I've just been going to work, sleeping, work again.

Nurse, community care, female, age 51–64

My partner is working interstate for several months, so this has meant living alone for the second lockdown in Victoria. We are both doctors, so we understand that's part of it all, but it's really hard not to be able to see each other because of the restrictions and border closures. I also have a five-month-old nephew, who I have only met once, and a brother who lives in the United States. I worry about him a lot.

Junior doctor, obstetrics, female, age 20–30

I have had to contend with the additional burden of having family interstate including my children, the non-COVID related deaths of two aunties, and parents that I care for in my own home also. This has increased my anxiety exponentially.

Nurse, pathology, female, age 51–64

Struggling without being able to see my 17-year-old son, who entered the army just as the COVID-19 restrictions happened. It has nearly been six months since I have been able to see him, and with travel not opening interstate anytime soon, this is affecting both our mental health, terrible on some days.

Allied health practitioner, female, age 41–50

I need the borders open—to visit my daughter—as then I will be refreshed and able to provide the utmost care to my clients.

Nurse, surgical, female, age 51–64

It may not be work related, but the fact I have only seen my four-month-old grandchild face-to-face three times is heartbreaking. I have not been able to support my daughter becoming a mother as I would have liked.

Nurse, community care, female, age 51–64

I feel sad not being able to touch or hug people if they are sad or need comfort. I feel tired and sad that I cannot visit my elderly parents in aged care.

Radiographer, medical specialty, female, age 41–50

> The lockdown between states has been a challenge when elderly parents live in another state.
>
> *Senior doctor, medical specialty, female, age 51–64*

> My father [in aged care] is not able to communicate on the phone and no-one can visit, which is devastating. My mother-in-law has had to deal with this largely on her own because her five children all live interstate or in a hot spot. We are a few hours' drive away and can only listen to her crying on the phone, because to visit her would mean a two-week quarantine away from our two young children.
>
> *Speech pathologist, community care, female, age 31–40*

> For more than three months I was only able to visit my parent by standing on the roadway down below her room's window and talking via the phone.
>
> *Nurse, palliative care, female, age 51–64*

Healthcare workers with family overseas told us about the dual distress of being separated from loved ones—with no end in sight—and worrying about the safety of family in countries with high rates of death from COVID-19.

> What is happening in other countries, to family overseas, has a significant impact on our mental health.
>
> *Nurse, obstetrics, female, age 41–50*

> My family all live overseas. I was more worried about them than myself, as I would be unable to go and see them if anything happened.
>
> *Nurse, research, female, age 51–64*

> My parents live overseas. My father passed away in April, from the consequences of COVID-19. I was unable to travel. My mother is now going through a severe depression, needs to move house, and again I am unable to travel.
>
> *Administrative worker, medical specialty, male, age 51–64*

> The inability to travel to the United Kingdom to spend time with my mother, who has a terminal illness, is a cause of intermittent, significant stress.
>
> *Senior doctor, paediatrics, female, age 41–50*

> Wishing and hoping that the pandemic will be over, and the border could re-open, so that I could meet my family. I miss them a lot and I have not met them for more than a year.
>
> *Nurse, intensive care, female, age 31–40*

> The fear that this is going to go on for a few years is deeply disturbing. I want to see my daughter, grandchildren, and mum all of whom live in New

> Zealand. And yet it looks highly likely that it will be a very long time until I can go there again. This saddens me greatly.
>
> *Nurse, medical specialty, male, age 51–64*

> I feel desperate as my close family resides overseas and I can't visit them for an uncertain time.
>
> *Senior doctor, paediatrics, female, age 41–50*

> Not being able to visit family in the UK for which I had planned with my long service leave.
>
> *Nurse, emergency department, female, age 51–64*

> Unique stress of being unable to bring elderly parents from overseas to keep them safe, due to visa restrictions, or visit them quickly in time of need due to lack of flights and permissions.
>
> *Senior doctor, medical specialty, male, age 41–50*

> It's really difficult being international and not knowing when you'll be able to see your family again.
>
> *Junior doctor, female, age 20–30*

Bereavement

Healthcare workers who had lost family and friends during the pandemic told us about the heartbreak caused by restrictions on the ability to travel, the size of funerals, and contact with family after the death of a loved one.

> Not being able to have a funeral for my nephew who died a horrific death from cancer was abysmal.
>
> *Allied health practitioner, dental care, female, age 51–64*

> My parents and family were unable to grieve together and normally after the death of a very close family member during lockdown.
>
> *Senior doctor, anaesthetics, female, age 41–50*

> I have just lost my mother in aged care of a natural death. Due to myself coming in contact with a positive COVID patient I was banned from seeing my dying mum. I tested negative twice, wore full PPE, and as per infection control was not required to quarantine and continued to work. My precious mother requested for me to be with her but she passed away alone. This has impacted me, as I did not get the support I needed. I have given my all to other sick patients and was forbidden from my own flesh and blood.
>
> *Nurse, community care, female, age 51–64*

My mother died, and I was not allowed to visit my sister to grieve, whilst partners not living together were allowed to catch up whenever they wanted to.

Psychologist, community care, female, age 41–50

The hardest challenge was not being allowed to visit my sick mother in hospital where she died on the third day of admission.

Occupational therapist, community care, female, age 51–64

My mum passed away during the pandemic. Her funeral of ten people in attendance was so sterile it hurts, and my children could not attend. I haven't seen my son who lives rurally, and my daughter who lives interstate, due to the lockdowns. It is really, really hard!

Nurse, hospital-based, female, age 41–50

I lost my grandfather in New Zealand during this time. Not being able to go home to say goodbye or attend the funeral will likely have long-term emotional implications for myself and my family.

Nurse, medical specialty, female, age 31–40

There has been little acknowledgement of the immigrants who have lost close family that were living overseas, but were unable to travel to a funeral or other gathering. We hear most about people who can't get back into Australia. My mum overseas died from COVID … I couldn't get there.

Senior doctor, medical specialty, male, age 51–64

With elderly family members and friends, maintaining the social connection has been difficult. We have had two deaths and have not been able to visit and attend funerals. We don't get this time back.

Allied health practitioner, medical specialty, female, age 51–64

My personal experience of my mum's death has affected how seriously I take the impact of this pandemic. It's hard to know whether it's COVID or grief that impacts how I'm coping.

Nurse, medical specialty, female, age 51–64

Loneliness, living alone, and isolation

Healthcare workers, particularly those who lived alone, described the burden of loneliness. The disruption to social activity caused by lockdown restrictions was one contributor to loneliness; another was self-imposed isolation due to the possible risk of infection they posed to others.

As a single person living alone, feeling like no-one cares. Not knowing who to talk to.

Phlebotomist, pathology, female, age 51–64

Living alone is the hardest. Not being able to see my parents in particular.

Nurse, hospital aged care, female, age 51–64

I want to stop feeling so lonely and isolated.

Junior doctor, general medicine, male, age 20–30

As I live alone, at times it felt very isolating, particularly as my family are in New South Wales and most of my friends in Victoria are outside my five-kilometre radius.

Junior doctor, female, age 31–40

Living alone and working alone (telehealth from home) increased feelings of isolation and loneliness.

Speech pathologist, medical specialty, female, age 41–50

Loneliness. I live alone and haven't seen my family in nearly a year due to them living outside the city.

Nurse, general medicine, male, age 20–30

Separated just before the pandemic so quite isolated at home as a single person.

Junior doctor, medical specialty, male, age 41–50

I am single and have found the lack of contact with my friends and family has been distressing at times. I am very independent and like my own company but have been surprised how much the isolation has affected me.

Nurse, community care, female, age 65–70

I am currently single, so not having a partner available to chat to has been difficult. The social isolation has also been hard.

Nurse, emergency department, female, age 41–50

Social isolation. Being single, and living alone, means I haven't seen a single person without masks in six weeks.

Junior doctor, medical specialty, female, age 31–40

Very challenging living alone and with my partner interstate.

Senior doctor, medical specialty, female, age 41–50

> Communication and contact: I live alone and just having a coffee with a friend or colleague would boost my morale.
>
> *Nurse, surgical, female, age 51–64*

> I have felt lonely at times as my husband has had to change his hours of work to avoid busy travel periods which leaves me alone for long periods during the week. I am missing the social connection and Zoom has lost a lot of its novelty when you spend your whole working day on it!
>
> *Speech pathologist, community care, female, age 51–64*

> I have seen friends on one occasion since March—who were also doctors—and we met up outdoors when the restrictions were eased. I have essentially become isolated because everyone else has been too concerned to meet up with me due to my job, even during safer periods.
>
> *Senior doctor, respiratory medicine, female, age 31–40*

> I am very lonely living alone. I lost my dog this year and my brother passed away. At first, I felt guilty I was not doing COVID clinics but being immunosuppressed, I couldn't. I spoke to my son about my death. I have isolated myself as my contacts don't understand or ask about the risk we face with each patient, not knowing if they are positive … I really just want to stay home, I'm tired, lonely and sad and even writing this makes me feel guilty.
>
> *Nurse, female, age 51–64*

Some healthcare workers told us that they wished that the concept of a "social bubble" had been adopted sooner in Australia.

> I feel the social needs of single people who live alone have been severely impacted in Victoria's restrictions.
>
> *Junior doctor, medical specialty, female, age 31–40*

> Having a social bubble, so that friends can debrief, makes a massive difference, especially because COVID means I didn't see any family for six months and counting!
>
> *Nurse, intensive care, female, age 20–30*

> Allow people who live on their own to see one other household.
>
> *General practitioner, female, age 41–50*

> I think this single social bubble is important and probably should have come in sooner. It's difficult living alone and not seeing friends or family.
>
> *Junior doctor, surgical, female, age 20–30*

Alone at work

Even work could be a lonely place, with the team camaraderie of meal breaks and causal interactions no longer available due to working from home or social-distancing and closure of tearooms at work.

> It has been difficult as I am a people person and enjoy the company of my fellow workers. I think it would be helpful to have more Zoom meetings for those working at home where we could just have a cuppa and chat over morning/afternoon tea.
>
> *Administrative worker, community care, female, age 51–64*

> The sexism, racism and homophobia that can usually be shrugged off or diluted with positive social interactions with family and friends has been amplified, since work colleagues are basically the only people we're interacting with consistently. It is horrible and lonely.
>
> *Nurse, research, female, age 31–40*

> I also now appreciate the value of team coffee breaks for mental health and human connection. Now that we can't even sit in the same room together, I feel very disconnected.
>
> *Junior doctor, medical specialty, female, age 31–40*

> Having to eat in isolation at work is really hard.
>
> *Nurse, community care, female, age 41–50*

> Working night duty adds another dimension to my stress—feeling isolated from the main workforce, from experts, and from communication … everything seems to be aimed at daytime workers.
>
> *Disability support worker, hospital aged care, female, age 51–64*

> As many people worked from home early on, the environment became very stark and isolating so you felt "everyone had run for cover" and you were left to hold the ground.
>
> *Occupational therapist, palliative care, female, age 65–70*

> It was very isolating when all the allied health/other staff left. It would have been great to have some contact from someone to say "we are still thinking about you" (not just generic emails).
>
> *Nurse, respiratory medicine, female, age 41–50*

> COVID is isolating. If you are a healthcare worker, it is isolating as you view human interactions as dangerous and potentially infectious.
>
> *Nurse, surgical, female, age 41–50*

The strain on relationships

Few relationships escaped the pandemic unchanged. Some became closer, others more distant, while for some the changes were both good and bad.

> The impact on relationships is not black and white. My relationship with my partner is both stronger and more difficult.
>
> *Senior doctor, medical specialty, female, age 41–50*

Healthcare workers told us about the strain on their relationships and the ways in which this strain interfaced with other pandemic-related challenges.

> Living in a tiny house while my partner is working from home and a Year 12 [final school year] student is studying at home. No alone time, and my partner is very messy.
>
> *Support worker, aged care, female, age 51–64*

> The effect on my relationship with my partner. (I live alone—my partner does not live with me). Being more isolated than I already am.
>
> *Nurse, community care, female, age 51–64*

> Curfew and restrictions cause stress on family and partner and my dog. Curfew negatively affects the amount of support I am able to provide my family.
>
> *Administrative worker, general medicine, female, age 31–40*

> The impact of the pandemic response has been quite profound for me, in terms of leaving employment I had been in for more than 13 years, to work elsewhere in an entirely new area. And then to encounter marital concerns and the psychological distress of my children who have developed early concerns with sleeping and eating.
>
> *Physiotherapist, community care, female, age 41–50*

Some healthcare workers wrote about relationship breakdowns during the pandemic. Occasionally, these had a silver lining.

> I moved to Melbourne at the beginning of the pandemic, and then went through a relationship breakdown. This made the social isolation a lot more difficult than it otherwise would have been, if I had my usual networks available to me.
>
> *Nurse, community care, female, age 31–40*

> It ended a relationship due to that person's misunderstanding of my role and their risk of contracting the virus due to my exposure. On the bright side, I met someone better.
>
> *Nurse, general medicine, male, age 51–64*

Social connection and support

Alongside the experiences of social isolation, loneliness, grief, bereavement, and relationship struggles, healthcare workers told us about the supports that mattered during this time.

> Friends, family and social connection have been essential to mental wellbeing during COVID.
>
> *Junior doctor, medical specialty, female, age 20–30*

> My family was my saviour.
>
> *Nurse, surgical, female, age 51–64*

> Spend time with family as much as possible.
>
> *Junior doctor, intensive care, male, age 41–50*

> Stay in touch with the people you care about.
>
> *Student, surgical, male, age 20–30*

> Close contact with friends and family that understand the importance of health to both individuals and community.
>
> *Dentist, private practice, female, age 51–64*

> The most helpful supports have been from my family and close friends in health, as well as healthcare colleagues across the country and the world.
>
> *Social worker, hospital aged care, female, age 31–40*

> Very grateful for the many ways people can connect virtually with family and friends.
>
> *Medical photographer, medical imaging, female, age 41–50*

> I largely seek and receive support from my wife rather than the hospital or its staff.
>
> *Senior doctor, pathology, male, age 51–64*

> I am grateful to have a partner I like spending time with.
>
> *Nurse, emergency department, female, age 41–50*

> I have grown a lot closer to my husband which is a blessing.
>
> *Nurse, general medicine, female, age 20–30*

> Talking to my partner has been very therapeutic and healing.
>
> *Clinical scientist, surgical, female, age 31–40*

Due to the protracted lockdown restrictions in Melbourne, I have no social life and no family life, as my partner and family live overseas and interstate. I have only my work life and work friends, both of which have been soul-sustaining. Without this interaction and purpose, I would be lost in my own loneliness and isolation.

Senior doctor, medical specialty, female, age 31–40

When I told close friends and family that I wasn't okay, they all played a huge part in getting me through this and checking in and supporting me.

Nurse, general medicine, female, age 20–30

7

DISPENSABLE AND DISILLUSIONED

> I feel I have been forced to work in an unsafe manner due to lack of PPE. And as a result, I feel dispensable. My safety and welfare have been completely disregarded by management and the public health system. I have compared this feeling to what it must have felt like for young men being conscripted to war.
>
> *Nurse, emergency department, female, age 41–50*

Healthcare workers are at markedly higher risk of COVID-19 infection than people working in other occupations. Seven in ten healthcare workers who caught COVID-19 in the first year of the pandemic are reported to have acquired their infection at work. This chapter captures the betrayal, frustration, and fear felt by many healthcare workers in response to organisational lapses and delays in prioritising their health and safety. Key to their struggles to feel safe at work was the supply and fit-testing of Personal Protective Equipment (PPE). The theme of betrayal was also evident in healthcare workers' descriptions of their working conditions and problems with testing and contact tracing for COVID-19. Some healthcare workers wrote about feeling stigmatised and scapegoated for being a possible source of contagion at work and in the community. Those who contracted COVID-19 sometimes felt blamed rather than supported.

Disposable and dispensable

Powerful metaphors and descriptors were used by healthcare workers as they wrote about their pervading sense of being expendable at work.

> We are puppets to them.
>
> *Nurse, medical specialty, female, age 31–40*

DOI: 10.4324/9781003228394-7

> We're managed as if we're pawns in some middle manager's terrible game of chess.
>
> *Junior doctor, intensive care, male, age 20–30*

> We are just minions in their workforce and we are disposable.
>
> *Nurse, emergency department, female, age 41–50*

> I feel quite invisible, unimportant, taken for granted.
>
> *General practitioner, female, age 41–50*

> My mental health is the worst it's ever been but I feel like my workplace doesn't care about its employees and will work us until we burn out or kill ourselves, especially at the moment.
>
> *Nurse, intensive care, female, age 20–30*

> We need to work from the top and help management and executives do training in how to effectively communicate, make people feel valued and that we are more than just a number.
>
> *Nurse, emergency department, female, age 20–30*

The right to be safe at work

Healthcare workers, at all levels of seniority and from every profession, expressed a belief that their lives were not being protected by those in positions of power.

> We should be adopting a precautionary principle, not doing the least possible based on convenience and assuming "she'll be right mate", which is what Australia has been doing form the start.
>
> *Senior doctor, medical specialty, female, age 31–40*

> I am reluctant to work at my job without adequate protection, or without it being a priority to protect healthcare workers. The reactive response to biohazard risk. The numbers of staff infected in Australia. I feel expendable.
>
> *Disability support worker, community care, female, age 41–50*

> If there is not much evidence either way, such as with pregnant health workers, we should act now to reduce their exposure to the virus and protect them.
>
> *Nurse, medical specialty, female, age 31–40*

> Many of my nursing colleagues are very disillusioned about their expendability secondary to feeling they had to continually fight for adequate PPE until many nurses contracted COVID.
>
> *Nurse, medical specialty, female, age 41–50*

> Feeling secure in the workplace is paramount and this was not prioritised at the start.
>
> *Senior doctor, gynaecology, female, age 51–64*

> If there are more health care workers with COVID-19 per capita than other community members, then we are not being appropriately protected at work.
>
> *Student, female, age 31–40*

> We need to feel the government cares whether we are protected in our role as health care workers.
>
> *Senior doctor, anaesthetics, male, age 31–40*

Betrayed

Healthcare workers described their feelings of betrayal, of being unprotected at work, and of not being valued at work.

> Betrayed and unsupported by the leaders who are meant to protect me.
>
> *Senior doctor, surgical, male, age 41–50*

> Very cynical and let down by the government with its total abandonment and lack of respect and resources for general practice.
>
> *General practitioner, female, age 41–50*

> Betrayed by the government and the Department of Health: bitterly disappointed and betrayed.
>
> *Senior doctor, psychiatry, female, age 51–64*

> Mistrust with respect to people in leadership positions … Their failure has been comprehensive in protecting healthcare workers: nurses and doctors.
>
> *Senior doctor, anaesthetics, female, age 51–64*

> My health service promotes a principle of a "positive workplace" but their actions dishonour their pronounced intention, and mock their staff, with their failure to either recognise the obvious or by ignoring the evidence before them.
>
> *Nurse, residential aged care, male, age 51–64*

> Some medical administrators seem overtly hostile to the idea of keeping staff safe and it has resulted in massive outbreaks in multiple facilities across this state.
>
> *Junior doctor, intensive care, male, age 31–40*

> It's not so much the problems of dealing with the pandemic. I got into this business to look after people. The problem I feel is being treated like I'm expendable by the federal government and people running PPE guidelines.
>
> *Junior doctor, intensive care, male, age 31–40*

Healthcare workers also wrote about the consequences of being disillusioned.

> I had faith that my employers and hospital executives were looking out for us before this pandemic and I was prepared to step up. However, it's clear to me that they really are not looking out for their workers and don't have our best interests at heart, so I have not stepped up to care for COVID patients. I no longer believe that they are looking out for their employees and now feel disillusioned with the medical system and our government.
>
> *Senior doctor, anaesthetics, female, age 41–50*

> I am thinking of leaving the healthcare system. It became clear that I'm not important as an individual. I've also lost all good will towards the hospital. Prior to COVID I was able to act like an orderly or nurse when there was a shortage or stay late if there was an overrun. Since COVID, I've realised the hospital doesn't value me and I don't want to gift any good will to it.
>
> *Senior doctor, anaesthetics, gender not disclosed, age 41–50*

Protecting the workforce with personal protective equipment

Inadequate PPE exemplified healthcare workers' feelings of betrayal: they faced a long, uphill battle in obtaining appropriate PPE, being fit-tested for PPE, and receiving rest and hydration breaks while working in full PPE.

> Proper protection for healthcare workers is essential and still neglected.
>
> *Senior doctor, medical specialty, female, age 31–40*

> In February and March, all staff asked about wearing masks at work, but it wasn't supported by the organisation as they followed the Department of Health's recommendations. Later on, from July, we were all asked to wear masks at work. If wearing masks is effective, why weren't we allowed to wear them? That broke the trust and we felt disappointed.
>
> *Nurse, respiratory medicine, female, age 41–50*

> The local and national response has felt like healthcare workers, and in particular those with the least skills, are expendable. The lack of definitive provision of appropriate PPE, fit-testing, and blaming healthcare workers for having caught the virus outside of work have all left a bad feeling in many of us.
>
> *Senior doctor, anaesthetics, female, age 51–64*

> The stakes in our profession are usually high; the pandemic has heightened our awareness of those stakes. It is an important part of our professional responsibility to require of our respective employers appropriate, fit-for-purpose, safe arrangements to enable us to continue caring for our patients.
>
> *Paramedic, male, age 31–40*

PPE supply

Despite asking for adequate PPE from the earliest days of the pandemic, healthcare workers faced months of potentially life-threatening delays in obtaining basic surgical masks for all staff, and fit-tested N95 masks for those working with suspected or confirmed COVID-positive patients.

> PPE! For god's sake. We need it.
>
> *General practitioner, female, age 31–40*

> Staff should be provided with sufficient, and good quality, full PPE please.
>
> *Physiotherapist, emergency department, male, age 31–40*

> If we were well PPE'ed, I would feel much safer for myself as well as for the community I interact with.
>
> *Senior doctor, general medicine, male, age 41–50*

> The anxiety about not having enough PPE initially was terrible, and the stress was palpable for all staff. To think that we would have to work without adequate coverage for ourselves was awful.
>
> *Nurse, intensive care, female, age 31–40*

> I still do not believe I will have access to adequate PPE that will actually protect me from infection.
>
> *Junior doctor, intensive care, female, age 20–30*

> The public hospital administration would have happily thrown us frontline workers in front of the bus, with insufficient training and PPE.
>
> *Senior doctor, anaesthetics, female, age 41–50*

> I feel that many of us would have done better mentally if the hospital had gone to top-level PPE from the start, and pulled back if necessary. People on the COVID and suspected-COVID wards were stressed because they felt unprotected. Even now, the hospital is looking at winding things back because the "prevalence is low". Like a bunch of morons, they are going to have another outbreak, or a frontline worker will die before they take it seriously. This lack of seriousness is what causes people to be stressed.
>
> *Senior doctor, general medicine, male, age 41–50*

A common concern was that PPE was being supplied at a lower level than healthcare workers considered appropriate for the risks they were facing.

> At least half of the people you perform oropharyngeal and nasopharyngeal-swabs on will cough, or gag, very close to your face. This is stressful if you have to perform this all day with just a surgical mask.
>
> *Nurse, emergency department, female, age 41–50*

> An apron type gown is not OK for paramedics, who are often on hands-and-knees on the ground, managing patients with infection risk and aerosol-generating procedures. We need overalls and head coverage.
>
> *Paramedic, female, age 41–50*

> Yes, it is a respiratory condition. I don't even understand how some "experts" have been advocating that hand-washing and loose masks may be enough protection for healthcare workers. Just beyond understanding. Everyone should be wearing PAPRs [air-purifying respirators] and coveralls by now.
>
> *Senior doctor, intensive care, male, age 41–50*

They contrasted the response to COVID-19 with responses to other infectious diseases, and other industries, where appropriate protection was readily available.

> Please supply N95 masks! Before the pandemic, N95s were used for influenza A and B, active chickenpox, and shingles. It's foolish to say the surgical mask is just as good as N95 while caring for the suspected COVID patients. Healthcare workers are not bulletproof!
>
> *Nurse, medical specialty, female, age 41–50*

> When I was working in infectious diseases during the Ebola outbreak (and we were the state-receiving centre for possible cases), the leadership from consultants and infection control was outstanding. The plan regarding isolation, management, and PPE was crystal clear. It made an enormous difference to how comfortable I felt working there. With COVID, the message changes constantly and—honestly—the decisions around what PPE we need to use seem to be based on what's available and not.
>
> *Junior doctor, emergency department, female, age 31–40*

> Police and firefighters are given a better quality of PPE—white coveralls, N95 masks, long cuff gloves—than doctors and nurses.
>
> *Junior doctor, intensive care, male, age 31–40*

Several healthcare workers described being mocked or accused of "overreacting" by managers when they asked to wear masks early in the pandemic.

> Management initially jeered at a fellow colleague who suggested mask-wearing during the early onset of COVID. They laughed at him and said that "it was a Chinese thing to wear masks".
>
> *Nurse, surgical, female, age 41–50*

> Early in the pandemic, private hospital employees were told not to wear masks—not even allowed to bring in their own to wear—despite those in public hospitals being allowed to do so.
>
> *Senior doctor, anaesthetics, female, age 41–50*

> For healthcare workers who were feeling anxious, PPE should have been made easily available. They should not have felt condemned for wanting to protect themselves.
>
> *Junior doctor, medical specialty, female, age 31–40*

> I felt, quite early on in the pandemic, that we should all be wearing masks. I could see back in March that there was a shortage of masks, so I spoke to my boss about buying my own masks to wear at work. I was told that "it would not be a good look". I wore one anyway, and I found that some of my colleagues felt the same, and started wearing a mask too. I found that my patients felt safer when I wore the mask. However, I also felt judgement from others, like I was "overreacting". I guess the main challenge for me has been wanting PPE and infection control measures put in place much sooner, and feeling anxious until they were finally put in place.
>
> *Radiographer, emergency department, female, age 41–50*

Restricting and limiting PPE use

Even when there was PPE available, healthcare workers told us about restrictions on its use.

> As healthcare workers, we should be provided with sufficient PPE where we do not have to reuse a disposable face shield for months.
>
> *Nurse, medical specialty, female, age 31–40*

> Having enough PPE to use (not re-using a mask all day when they have previously been changed for each patient), not having adequate breaks because the PPE cannot be discarded and only one set is available per shift, and not having alternative well-fitting masks are a concern.
>
> *Senior doctor, anaesthetics, female, age 41–50*

> Using single-use PPE such as gowns between patients—which is our practice at a big hospital during the pandemic—goes against the principles of

infection control that we were taught in university. I have felt that changing the rules to apply to the pandemic, and using gowns between patients, enhances the spread of infection.

Nurse, emergency department, male, age 31–40

Up-to-date information would have been good coming from the network I work in. Not once did we have any information from infection-control. PPE availability is related to money available, not safety requirements.

Nurse, emergency department, female, age 51–64

Department of Health guidelines were poor, especially for frontline workers and especially when community transmission increased. Essentially this workforce is expendable due to Safer Care Victoria's lack of admission of airborne transmission and rationing of PPE at commencement of the second wave.

Nurse, emergency department, female, age 31–40

I am an anaesthetist, and can afford increased levels of protective gear, or to not work if I choose. The nursing teams I work with don't have that luxury. I feel that this pandemic has widened the gap between the haves and the have-nots. There are issues of powerlessness, and being made to work whilst not feeling safe.

Senior doctor, anaesthetics, female, age 41–50

We are all tired, stressed and "saving" PPE (by wearing masks longer than we should). Some doctors are sanitising their gloves. I think this is all due to the fact that we feel PPE is "rationed".

Nurse, general practice, female, age 51–64

Tasks in the isolation rooms are cohorted together to minimise PPE usage.

Nurse, surgical, female, age 31–40

Working in a surgical ward I have felt as though we are the last priority in the context of COVID-19 which I understand, but this has impacted my mental health. We were one of the last areas that were able to wear surgical masks on the floor. Prior to mandatory PPE across all clinical and non-clinical areas of the hospital, it was only "high risk" areas that were provided with PPE. Patients from the intensive care unit and emergency department were escorted to the ward by nurses in full PPE, when the surgical masks on our ward were literally locked up. I didn't feel safe and, when myself and others voiced this, our concerns were dismissed by infection control. I understand that there was a shortage of PPE.

Nurse, surgical, female, age 20–30

PPE design and fit-testing

Mask fit-testing is a procedure that matches an N95 (or P2) mask with the face shape and size of the wearer, to ensure maximum protection. If a mask doesn't fit properly, the healthcare worker is at risk of breathing in airborne virus particles. Throughout the first and second waves of the pandemic, healthcare workers in Australia cared for COVID-positive patients without the protection of mandatory fit-testing of masks.

> All staff should have mask-fittings. This would reduce stress knowing we are best protected.
>
> *Nurse, intensive care, female, age 51–64*

> Lack of N95 fit-testing is making me feel uneasy and stressed.
>
> *Senior doctor, medical specialty, female, age 31–40*

> Some hospitals still don't fit-test. I know I have failed the fit-test, but would still be required to perform aerosol generating procedures in affected patients anyway.
>
> *Senior doctor, anaesthetics, female, age 41–50*

> We are to this day fighting against hospital administrators to be allowed to get fit-tested for N95 masks that actually fit.
>
> *Senior doctor, anaesthetics, female, age 41–50*

> Not implementing the same respiratory PPE regimes, including fit-testing, for staff in hospital as in other industries with respiratory risks is disgusting.
>
> *Senior doctor, intensive care, male, age 41–50*

> Dentistry is such a high aerosol generating industry. It would be great for hospital and health executives to listen when staff are supplied with PPE that is not fit for purpose. To constantly be fobbed off is so disrespectful.
>
> *Oral health therapist, community care, female, age 31–40*

PPE wearing

While most healthcare workers welcomed the protection offered by PPE, they drew attention to the challenges of wearing PPE, including difficulties communicating, regulating body temperature, staying hydrated, attending to patient care, and managing fatigue. Again, they felt that there was little acknowledgement—or accommodation—from their organisations in response to these new challenges.

PPE is the pits. Exhausting to work in physically, and from a communicative point of view between staff and patients.

Physiotherapist, emergency department, female, age 41–50

I find it really hard working in PPE all the time as our work area is too hot and uncomfortable.

Clinical scientist, pathology, female, age 51–64

Face shields get in the way while assisting with continence care, forcing you to take odd positions while bending over, giving a personal wash, and dressing patients.

Nurse, aged care, female, age 51–64

It is such misery to know that you'll end up having to wear PPE for ten-plus hours, not being able to drink water or use the toilet as much as you'd like, and also being worried about potential exposure.

Nurse, intensive care, female, age 31–40

It's difficult not having easy access to fresh air during our breaks. It's really stifling wearing a mask all day!

Occupational therapist, community care, female, age 31–40

The time taken to don and doff PPE means seeing each patient takes quite a bit longer, and it is harder to keep on top of paperwork between patients.

Junior doctor, emergency department, female, age 31–40

I tend to get more irritable wearing PPE, especially when trying to learn new electronic medical record systems.

Nurse, perioperative care, female, age 41–50

Just the hearing thing with PPE. It really impacts communication which affects handover, which is identified in healthcare as a potential risk.

Physiotherapist, medical specialty, female, age 51–64

Wearing masks all the working week has become incredibly stressful. It was difficult to speak and understand people and the masks were incredibly uncomfortable. It can be hard to get to know new staff with all the PPE.

Nurse, respiratory medicine, female, age 31–40

Wearing the PPE makes it hard to bond with other staff and reduces the enjoyment of work significantly.

Senior doctor, respiratory medicine, male, age 41–50

> Wearing a face shield and mask all shift feels like it is contributing to my tiredness.
>
> *Nurse, discharge planning, female, age 41–50*

> I also became fatigued through extra concentration to the PPE in protecting myself.
>
> *Clinical scientist, infectious diseases, female, age 51–64*

> The importance of nursing staff keeping well hydrated and taking the time to go to the toilet appropriately. Sometimes you're in full PPE for eight to ten hours and go home feeling dehydrated as no drinks are allowed on the floor.
>
> *Nurse, emergency department, female, age 51–64*

> When wearing face masks and shields, you tend to drink far less and become dehydrated. It is not easy to stop and get a drink of water let alone a decent meal during an outbreak.
>
> *Nurse, residential aged care, female, age 41–50*

Healthcare workers made a number of recommendations for workplace accommodations that would improve their ability to work safely and effectively while wearing full-PPE.

> Allow free parking for staff and supply appropriate areas for meal breaks instead of encouraging people to sit in their cars for their breaks, while trying to don and doff within the limited time frame.
>
> *Nurse, emergency department, female, age 31–40*

> Working in PPE creates a level of inefficiency that means I can only perform at about 75 percent of my usual capacity. After four hours in PPE, I become so fatigued that I start to have trouble making decisions and can see my risk of making mistakes start to increase. Shorter shifts with adequate staff to allow breaks would help to address this, but these are not provided by hospital management.
>
> *Senior doctor, emergency department, female, age 41–50*

COVID-19 testing

Healthcare workers were acutely aware of their risk of contracting COVID-19 and were keen to ensure that any testing and contact tracing system was effective and efficient. At the same time, they were aware of the burden on patients and colleagues when they needed to take time off to be tested for symptoms such as fever, cough, headache, runny nose, or sore throat, which could indicate COVID-19, but were more commonly due to simple colds or allergies.

> The introduction of priority testing significantly decreased my stress levels, knowing I would have minimal time off waiting for a swab result when I was concerned about the impact of being quarantined on my patients and colleagues. Having to cancel and rearrange clinics of 60-plus patients per day, and theatre lists for urgent patients, is extremely stressful as a clinician. It impacts patients, their extended families, patients' employers, community supports and dependents, and creates work for countless other staff. The knock-on effects are huge. The concerns about the effect of having time off at short notice—and the even bigger concerns about the risk of not taking time off and spreading COVID—have both been stressful. If rapid testing comes in as suggested that will help immensely.
>
> *Senior doctor, surgical, female, age 31–40*

> I think all front-line workers should have a fortnightly test for screening and to reduce anxiety that they could be the asymptomatic spreader to family or colleagues.
>
> *Nurse, emergency department, female, age 41–50*

Healthcare workers believed that a consistent, integrated system for testing and contact tracing would improve our ability to contain the virus.

> Contact tracing needs to be actioned in all hospitals where visitors and staff take a photo of a QR code, do a survey, then print out a docket and stick it on yourself with a date so it can be better managed. Some hospitals already have this but mine doesn't.
>
> *Support worker, emergency department, male, age 31–40*

> It has been a bit anxiety provoking to see how chaotic the contact tracing of my COVID positive colleague was—by August I thought it would be working—and how easily small errors can lead to big spread in a hospital.
>
> *Senior doctor, anaesthetics, female, age 51–64*

> There was a lack of communication between contact tracing, pathology, and the clearance centre. No-one knew what anyone else was up to. I was told they would get back to me, but then no-one got back to me. I had to follow it up myself. Some members of the Department of Health team give information that is wrong, or not up to date, which adds to the confusion.
>
> *Nurse, community care, female, age 31–40*

COVID-19 infection

Thousands of healthcare workers were infected with COVID-19 during the second wave of the pandemic in Australia. Healthcare workers voiced concern about the high numbers of infections, the fact that most were workplace-acquired, and the potential long-term health consequences.

> The COVID infection rate in health care workers is alarmingly high.
>
> *Senior doctor, medical specialty, male, age 51–64*

> I am looking after some patients who contracted COVID through their hospital work after being given inadequate PPE at a time when there was obvious risk (the catchment area was hotspot-ridden, and the risk of asymptomatic transmission risk was well known by that stage). They have significant complications, and their well-being will be affected for a long time due to the failure of this institution to protect their staff.
>
> *General practitioner, female, age 31–40*

For healthcare workers infected with COVID-19, their anguish is palpable in their accounts of their own illness as well as the repercussions for their families.

> When I got told I was positive from an asymptomatic test, my world changed so fast. Being alone, wondering if you were going to deteriorate, wondering if you were ever doing to see your family again, hold your children, hug your parents and sister. My husband couldn't even console me when I was told, because I knew the risks.
>
> *Nurse, surgical, female, age 31–40*

> I contracted COVID at work and infected my husband and daughter.
>
> *Occupational therapist, hospital aged care, female, age 31–40*

> We are not expendable, and we have families that are affected by the consequences of us being infected with COVID. Our concerns are genuine.
>
> *Nurse, community care, female, age 41–50*

> I was infected with COVID-19 on placement and was very unwell. I am disappointed that the university would put students at risk, dismiss their concerns, and not express any empathy for their students.
>
> *Student, respiratory medicine, female, age 20–30*

> I felt very unsupported by the medical school when I was unwell with COVID-19 and made to feel like it was my fault, or that it was the result of community transmission, when it definitely was not.
>
> *Medical student, respiratory medicine, female, age 20–30*

> It was devastating spreading COVID to my partner and watching him get sick too.
>
> *Nurse, emergency department, female, age 31–40*

> My pregnant daughter who is a frontline nurse caught COVID at 17 weeks' pregnancy and I was fearful she and the baby would die. She passed COVID to my son also and I feared he would not survive either. In turn, my husband and I were quarantined whilst fretting about our child and grandchild who were COVID positive. My son's school was also placed in lockdown, so the knock-on effect has been astonishing and awful.
>
> *Nurse, palliative care, female, age 51–64*

> I think we are worried about the long-term effects as both of us still have side effects from the virus.
>
> *Nurse, casual pool, female, age 51–64*

The need for support for healthcare workers infected with COVID-19 through their recovery, and in returning to work, was important, as was the recognition that COVID-19 infection was a workplace safety issue.

> I was in quarantine after contracting the virus. The Hotels for Heroes program was really good. I had someone calling me every day to make sure I was feeling okay, and she would call me twice a day on the days where I was really unwell. I think there should be more ongoing support for people who recover from the virus.
>
> *Nurse, hospital aged care, female, age 20–30*

> My workplace was supportive: daily contact to make sure I was OK, and to arrange for things I needed.
>
> *Nurse, casual pool, male, age 20–30*

> I felt like I was coping well, until I had to completely isolate from my family. That took a great emotional toll on me and it has been a struggle for me to return to work since.
>
> *Nurse, intensive care, female, age 20–30*

> As a healthcare worker who contracted COVID-19, on return, we are treated differently in that our colleagues unintentionally avoid us.
>
> *Radiographer, emergency department, female, age 20–30*

> Some staff felt pressured to return back to work after they have been unwell with COVID-19.
>
> *Nurse, COVID-screening clinic, age 20–30*

> I believe positive staff could have been given more assistance and acknowledgement for their hard work and contracting the virus on the job.
>
> *Nurse, surgical, female, age 31–40*

> We need paid sick leave for days off due to COVID-testing and [becoming] COVID-positive workers, as it is more than likely that staff have picked it up at work. Health services should not be making it a battle for staff to claim these benefits they should be entitled to.
>
> *Nurse, emergency department, female, age 20–30*

> Having secure access to WorkCover [workers compensation] if healthcare workers become infected with COVID is very important.
>
> *Senior doctor, surgical, female, age 41–50*

> Wellbeing is directly related to our perception of safety. So far very little has been done to reassure us of our safety. Most clinicians have to deal with COVID daily. To then have to fight for our basic rights with institutions that are supposed to guarantee our safety is a waste of time and effort and adds to clinician stress and takes away from patient care. The total waste of our six month lead time from the start of this pandemic back in January is a clear example of how it's hard for clinicians to have faith in the system. The systems failures contribute significantly to healthcare worker burnout, anxiety and emotional despair. Not to mention there is also a financial cost to many clinicians that are not covered under the current government financial rebate schemes like Jobkeeper. Government financial support specific to healthcare workers is crucial to wellbeing. Things like removing the burden of proof for Workcover in the middle of a pandemic is just common sense that healthcare workers should not have to waste time fighting for and worrying about.
>
> *Senior doctor, emergency department, female, age 31–40*

Scapegoating and shame

Many healthcare workers discussed the scapegoating and stigma associated with the spread of the virus. The "blame game" they write about occurred in both workplace and community settings, leading many to feel that they were under siege in both spheres of their lives.

> I still feel that there is a blame associated with the virus, through statements like "all transmission in Victoria can be traced back to one family in hotel quarantine". I can't help but think this is unfair. Do this family now have to deal with the hundreds of aged care deaths?
>
> *Nurse, female, age 41–50*

> Remove the blame from healthcare workers. We work in a high-risk environment. Admittedly we are human and can make mistakes, but do not cast blame when we get sick.
>
> *Radiographer, emergency department, female, age 31–40*

> The blame game is counterproductive. We are all human and the virus is highly contagious, so errors are bound to occur.
>
> *Junior doctor, emergency department, male, age 31–40*

> Stop blaming healthcare workers who become positive rather than supporting them, assuming they got it from community transmission despite them working on hot [COVID-19] wards four days a week.
>
> *Nurse, casual pool, female, age 20–30*

> The hardest part of the COVID pandemic is when colleagues contracted the disease. It was upsetting to hear senior staff pass the blame on incorrect PPE adherence when all staff have been diligent about protecting themselves.
>
> *Nurse, general medicine, female, age 20–30*

> I have felt a lot of negative responses to how staff have felt punished, blamed or talked down to by hospital executive. The "healthcare heroes" doesn't really ring true in the hospital.
>
> *Junior doctor, medical specialty, female, age 20–30*

> My workplace ignores the risks we face and puts it back on us: "It's your responsibility to socially distance". On a ward full of staff!
>
> *Nurse, maternity, female, age 41–50*

> I think there should be more dialogue around the fact that using PPE all the time is exhausting, and if you do catch COVID it is not your fault and you should feel no guilt.
>
> *Student, infectious diseases, female, age 20–30*

Community perceptions and blaming healthcare workers

We heard that healthcare workers were, on the one hand, supported by the community and, on the other hand, seen as potentially spreading the virus.

> Some public are openly grateful and appreciative, but a majority (locally for me anyway) are worried about our presence in the public and fear that we are contagious. For example, our management advised us to stop wearing our scrubs in public (i.e., getting petrol or food on the way home) because of the risk to us.
>
> *Nurse, emergency department, female, age 20–30*

> Community opinion that we will give them the virus if they come near us can be isolating. You feel like you are unable to disclose your job to others.
>
> *Nurse, intensive care, female, age 20–30*

When I wore scrubs outside a COVID area, I could see people were worried being around me.

Senior doctor, respiratory medicine, male, age 41–50

Our kids' piano and Chinese tutors cancelled their lessons before their peers. I couldn't help but think it was because we were health care workers.

Senior doctor, anaesthetics, female, age 41–50

Our relationships with friends and family have been strained, people cross the street when they see us walking in our scrubs, people abuse us in supermarkets if we are there in our scrubs before work.

Nurse, infectious diseases, female, age 20–30

The saddest part is being avoided by extended family and friends, thanks to the media implicating that health workers were being infected in the community, making it seem that we were irresponsible!

Allied health practitioner, rehabilitation, female, age 51–64

I constantly felt discriminated against by the public that I was high-risk. I've been caring for patients with influenza, norovirus, and tuberculosis prior to this pandemic and the public had no concerns.

Nurse, emergency department, female, age 20–30

Feeling valued from a distance, but also ostracised by the community given community fears of catching COVID-19.

General practitioner, female, age 31–40

8

OVERWORK, BURNOUT, AND RESIGNATION

> After nearly ten years of enthusiastically nursing, this pandemic has broken me, as it has a lot of others. I have sacrificed my mental health, physical health, and close relationships. My expenses have increased, and I have had to decrease my work hours due to burnout. While I could not quit working, I would technically be better off financially supported by the government staying home than what I earn literally killing myself to help people through this. This has destroyed bedside nursing for me and for the sake of my mental health I will have to leave the field once I mentally accept that I can no longer help others because no one helped us when we needed it.
>
> *Nurse, hospital aged care, female, age 20–30*

During the pandemic, rates of burnout, fatigue, anxiety, and depression among healthcare workers surged. Increased demand on services, relentless and rapid changes to working roles and responsibilities, and chronic understaffing, combined to contribute to higher workloads, longer working hours, and more stress for many healthcare workers. In this chapter we present healthcare workers' descriptions of overwork and burnout, and the factors that contributed to these experiences. Their stories illustrate the immense demands placed on individual healthcare workers and how these pressures contributed to a sense of helplessness and resignation. Healthcare workers—especially those in positions with less power or autonomy—frequently described feeling let down and unsupported in their workplace. Indeed, some felt driven to leave their profession.

DOI: 10.4324/9781003228394-8

Workload

Healthcare workers told us that their already considerable workloads increased dramatically after the onset of the pandemic because of additional duties and stressors, the increasing complexity of patient admissions, and the increasing number of colleagues who were required to take sick leave.

> The added extra duties have put a real strain on our work environment. Doing observations on residents every day, COVID screening, screening of staff and residents' families, more paperwork. It's impossible to maintain social distancing in this field of work. Wearing masks and eye googles all shift is a real drainer. Dementia patients have got no idea what you are saying. This job has changed, and certainly not for the better. Myself and my colleagues are very stressed with the extra workload on top of what was already a huge workload working in aged care.
>
> *Nurse, hospital aged care, female, age 31–40*

> I felt bullied into taking extra shifts.
>
> *Nurse, hospital aged care, female, age 51–64*

> The added complexity and volume of work in a short time is exhausting to keep up with.
>
> *Paramedic, female, age 51–64*

> I had to increase my on-call workload and that means staying all weekend at a hotel close to the hospital.
>
> *Senior doctor, anaesthetics, female, age 41–50*

> I was feeling burnt out by the issues and challenges posed by mental health concerns among patients even before the pandemic. Now with the pandemic, work conditions are much worse. GPs are expected to be workhorses. In order to maintain our income and continue to provide excellent levels of care we are expected to work twice as hard with little support.
>
> *General practitioner, female, age 51–64*

> We have faced more pressure for timelines of moving patients through ED. We offer on-call radiography services after-hours, and non-urgent imaging is routinely ordered overnight, rather than being held off to the morning. Interrupted sleep is very stressful.
>
> *Radiographer, hospital-based, female, age 51–64*

> The impact of being given extra work with no extra help has been huge. This has been my downfall.
>
> *Administrative worker, respiratory medicine, female, age 51–64*

Some healthcare workers expressed concern that the additional workload was not evenly distributed.

> It does feel unfair at times when my non-medical colleagues are able to work from home and those of us who have to be physically at work inevitably have to take in more of the "urgent" workload that they cannot address.
>
> *Junior doctor, female, age 31–40*

> As part of my position involved giving long-acting injections and face-to-face contact with high-risk mental health clients I was not able to work from home and thus the majority of face-to-face contact fell to myself and a few colleagues on my team. This had a huge impact on my health, both mental and physical. And although the extra work was recognised by my manager, there was nothing put in place to assist or reduce the workload.
>
> *Nurse, community care, female, age 51–64*

> I'm burnt out. Staff in the unit are trying to avoid working with COVID patients so a select few—including myself—are doing all the load.
>
> *Nurse, intensive care, male, age 20–30*

> We're all just exhausted. I was burnt out pre-pandemic and now feel so guilty about wanting to leave medicine. I will stay because I feel I need to, not because it's what's best for me.
>
> *Junior doctor, emergency department, female, age 31–40*

It was not just clinical tasks that took more time. Administrative tasks also increased in complexity.

> Because I don't work in a clinical capacity, people think that I am not affected but I have seen our workload in human resources double for each member of our team and we are really struggling to keep on top of new requirements from the Government and the hospital on top of our heavy workload. The impact on our department feels like we are drowning, and every priority is a priority, but no-one seems to understand the demands on us. Just because we are not clinical doesn't mean we don't feel the pressure like frontline workers.
>
> *Administrative worker, female, age 51–64*

In this context, healthcare workers called for flexibility in managers' expectations around performance targets and reporting requirements.

> I don't feel at this time we should be under the usual pressure to meet our key performance indicators for the sake of it.
>
> *Physiotherapist, community care, female, age 51–64*

We need more recognition that meeting targets and compliance activities isn't a sensible or necessary priority in the crisis context. Some of the reporting and compliance demands seem bizarre in the current context.

Social worker, community care, female, age 41–50

They concentrate on compliance to appropriate documentation and key performance indicators and forget about emotional wellbeing.

Paramedic, male, age 51–64

Being underpaid

Many healthcare workers, particularly nurses, noted that the increased workload was not accompanied by any additional recognition or remuneration.

Healthcare workers need better support and working conditions. It is not OK to work overtime and not be paid. That is not our fault and we do not have poor time management.

Nurse, surgical, female, age 31–40

I am the Contact Officer for my facility. I have been inundated with issues from all departments in our facility. I have done most of this on my own time, unpaid.

Nurse, hospital aged care, female, age 51–64

The level of unpaid and unappreciated overtime, problems associated with disorganisation within the system, and unrealistic expectations placed on clinical staff are the biggest burdens of the pandemic. It would be helpful to quantify the amount of unpaid overtime that is being completed and why.

Senior doctor, medical specialty, female, age 41–50

We still bulk bill [forego any fee beyond the government rebate] as patients are still vulnerable, but the length of time we spend per patient is longer. This adds to our stress. To see our usual workload means consulting for longer hours leading to more mental fatigue and burn out.

General practitioner, female, age 51–64

Staffing shortages

Healthcare workers shared their frustration about the lack of adequate staffing to meet the demands of the pandemic. The strain was felt in areas as diverse as aged care, emergency medicine, intensive care, mental health, and palliative care.

Health care in normal times is extremely stressful work. We need more staff, lower workloads, and more time to debrief.

Nurse, palliative care, female, age 41–50

> More staff are needed in most public health positions to cope with increased demand, especially in my field of mental health.
>
> *Psychologist, emergency department, female, age 41–50*

> Our teams would have benefited from increased resourcing to support staff during periods of additional training requirements, and also to emotionally support families of patients who were dealing with limited contact.
>
> *Physiotherapist, palliative care, female, age 51–64*

> Even if two or three of us were out of action for two weeks, there isn't enough staff to cover the gaps in the roster.
>
> *Administrative worker, female, age 31–40*

Healthcare workers described the bureaucratic hurdles they had to jump over when trying to ensure safe staffing levels. There was a perception that some managers cared more about their budgets than about patient care.

> It would be nice to call on additional mental health clinicians when we are really busy, without the need to go through the whole rigmarole of contacting the manager on call!
>
> *Nurse, emergency department, female, age 51–64*

> We need adequate personnel to manage—not having to beg for it each day.
>
> *Nurse, emergency department, female, age 51–64*

> I did not go into medicine to be denying care to patients who need it. If executives choose to continue to deny funding to staff the intensive care unit and emergency department appropriately, then they should be around on the floor to manage the consequences.
>
> *Junior doctor, intensive care, female, age 31–40*

> Regional hospitals with limited staff need help with staffing when rosters have deficits and locums can't travel. Hospital managers need to help make this happen and not scrimp on overtime for administrative tasks to be completed or for specialists to come from other hospitals.
>
> *Senior doctor, intensive care, male, age 41–50*

The staffing shortages, coupled with increased demands, left some healthcare workers feeling pressured to work unpaid overtime, or take on additional duties, to not let down colleagues or patients.

> People have to do extra work because we don't have enough staff in the emergency department to cope with the COVID leave.
>
> *Nurse, emergency department, female, age 51–64*

> It is exhausting that clinicians are just expected to do more, rather than hiring staff or replacing staff when they are away or leave.
>
> *Allied health practitioner, rehabilitation, female, age 31–40*

> Lack of staffing means lack of clinical care. I don't attend hospital-wide staff forums as I would like to because I don't want to take the time away from providing care to our patients which is my priority. The lack of backfill or staffing support makes this impossible, which is disappointing.
>
> *Physiotherapist, intensive care, female, age 31–40*

> I need a break from work, but I feel I can't as it will put too much strain on everyone else who is already working above capacity. Our area is starting to be concerning as a hotspot so I feel I can't abandon people in a time of need. We have no support or guidance from anyone.
>
> *General practitioner, female, age 41–50*

> When I was sick and needed a COVID swab, I felt so guilty that all of my work for those two days would fall to other members of the team or my patients would be disadvantaged. Having robust policies for how sick leave will be covered would make it so much easier to rest when you need to.
>
> *Junior doctor, palliative care, female, age 20–30*

> Being a frontline infectious diseases clinician makes it difficult to try and find time to take off without feeling guilty for my peers who then have to shoulder an increased load, and without feeling guilty for non-COVID activities which are part of my contract but are still placing demands on my time. We need protected time off without feeling guilty—but there is no redundancy in the system to allow this. I hardly know any of my infectious diseases colleagues who have had time off since February.
>
> *Senior doctor, infectious diseases, female, age 41–50*

> Overworked staff members in understaffed areas causes burnout and contributes to people calling in sick … causing MORE staff shortages, repeat and rinse.
>
> *Nurse, casual pool, female, age 20–30*

Staffing shortages also meant that healthcare workers worried that patient safety was being compromised—especially in aged care and on COVID wards.

> Not having extra staff is a constant source of anxiety. Worrying that because the resources are stretched so thin that you will make mistakes is terrifying.
>
> *Nurse, emergency department, female, age 20–30*

> Simple patient care tasks are made much more arduous and less timely, which has a great impact on our care and efficacy as a nurse. This means

> that the nurse-to-patient ratios during this time are unsafe. The need for more nurses is paramount for timely patient care to be maintained and delivered. It is almost impossible to do that when in potential COVID patients' rooms and trying to manage three to four critically unwell patients at a time. People's heath and lives are the factors that suffer most. Going home feeling like a terrible nurse every day because you are barely getting to each of the patients is an awful feeling on top of all other workplace pressures during COVID.
>
> *Nurse, emergency department, female, age 20–30*

The need for "guilt-free" time off

Healthcare workers spoke about needing time off, but felt reluctant or unable to take leave because of the additional burden on colleagues along with the inflexibility of health workplaces.

> I need to take leave, but I can't due to staffing levels being minimal all the time! COVID has just made it worse, and I can't go anywhere anyway.
>
> *Administrative worker, Aboriginal health, female, age 51–64*

> It seems hard to justify leaving my team to do all of the work. As a team leader, I worry for the wellbeing of my team. We're in this for the long haul, yet the burnout already feels so real.
>
> *Physiotherapist, intensive care, female, age 31–40*

> I have had no time off this year. What we need is to be able to take time off without feeling guilty that we will overload our peers in doing so. This is much more pronounced since COVID, but already existed pre-COVID.
>
> *Senior doctor, infectious diseases, female, age 41–50*

> The hospital is unforgiving when time off is needed.
>
> *Junior doctor, general medicine, female, age 41–50*

> Frontline workers who can't work from home need extra leave as stress in the healthcare workplace has escalated and is taking a toll.
>
> *Senior doctor, palliative care, female, age 41–50*

Healthcare workers reported that workplace changes were needed to ensure adequate time-off for healthcare workers to recharge, work through difficult emotions, and take care of their physical and mental health.

> COVID has been a massive burden on the mental health of all healthcare professionals. Yet at not one point have we had the chance to stop working or had the time to process all the things we have been through. We are

> expected to just keep working like we haven't just witnessed the tragedy of COVID.
>
> *Nurse, infectious diseases, female, age 20–30*

> It would have been helpful to offer leave, even just a few days, for health care workers who had worked on COVID wards at the end of their rotation. If I had had a break before starting a new rotation, I would have had time to process my experience and recover emotionally.
>
> *Pharmacist, hospital aged care, female, age 20–30*

> We have been lucky in getting the second wave under control, but doctors haven't taken much or any annual leave. In the department where I work, we are suffering mentally. We need strong support and direction to take some time off to maintain mental health, get away from the stress, refresh.
>
> *Senior doctor, medical specialty, female, age 51–64*

> I really feel that there needs to be a culture change in the workplace. If you are symptomatic for any illness, you must stay home. No more pushing through sickness because of guilt about leaving others with increased workloads. Instead, workplaces need to be better staffed to account for sick leave and recreational leave.
>
> *Speech pathologist, rehabilitation, female, age 31–40*

> We need better planning so that everyone can get some leave, as we all get more fatigued.
>
> *Junior doctor, emergency department, female, age 31–40*

> Managers need to make sure that health care workers are taking time to have leave even if there is nowhere to go.
>
> *Administrative worker, general medicine, female, age 51–64*

> I hope that this pandemic is changing the landscape for the future with regards to healthcare workers being encouraged to take sick leave when unwell.
>
> *Junior doctor, emergency department, female, age 20–30*

There was strong support for the idea of special pandemic leave or, at the very least, allowing staff greater flexibility around how and when they used their leave.

> I think staff should be allowed to stockpile leave if they want to and employees should plan for staff taking more leave next year and the year after and allow for that in staff planning.
>
> *Nurse, emergency department, female, age 41–50*

> At the end of this lockdown, clinics should close for a two-week period to give staff a break as we will be expected to go full steam ahead and get as many patients as possible into appointments after lockdown. This is when staff will feel the impact, as they have had no time for themselves, and the pressure will come from the hospital to get things back up and running to recoup lost revenue.
>
> *Administrative worker, medical specialty, female, age 51–64*

> Could the staff who have been on the frontline be given some extra annual leave after the pandemic to recoup and tend to themselves?
>
> *Psychologist, hospital aged care, female, age 51–64*

Relentless change

Constant changes at work, including changing conditions, processes, rules, and guidelines, added to the emotional and practical work for frontline healthcare workers.

> Changes in routine can be unsettling. There have literally been hundreds of changes to our workplace and practices. I have found it so draining mentally and physically.
>
> *Physiotherapist, emergency department, female, age 41–50*

> The day-to-day uncertainty, and constant changes of workloads and locations of work, is draining and anxiety-provoking.
>
> *Dietician, hospital aged care, female, age 41–50*

> We have changed things more than once, and this put a strain on education, equipment, and all staff. I have seen a lot of stressed people, throughout the hospital.
>
> *Nurse, intensive care, female, age 51–64*

> It is difficult to be a part-time health worker during COVID, as information changes frequently. It can be a full-time job to keep up. Mostly dealing with information overload, too many changes.
>
> *Senior doctor, palliative care, female, age 41–50*

> The Department of Health is adding to the stress of COVID by bringing in rules and regulations and changing what we do on a daily basis. Perhaps think ahead? This is stressful. Each day there is a new form, or process, or update, and we are fatigued from it.
>
> *Dietician, medical specialty, female, age 31–40*

During the pandemic, some large hospitals implemented major organisational changes including a switch from paper-based to electronic medical records, while also implementing COVID-related changes. Some nurses questioned the wisdom of trying to implement major change projects in the midst of a global pandemic.

> Implementing the electronic medical record at the height of the pandemic was cruel. It added a layer of extra stress in the workplace. No one listened to our concerns, and now the nurses are crying on shift, exhausted and frustrated, and patient care has been compromised. I felt like I went from a low maintenance nurse, to being very needy, at a time when everyone was struggling.
>
> *Nurse, intensive care, female, age 51–64*

> I wish the hospital wouldn't make so many changes that are not related to the COVID-19 pandemic because we cannot catch up with the constant change of information while trying to focus on the pandemic. It makes it harder when we already have poor communication.
>
> *Nurse, community care, female, age 31–40*

> Information changing has been stressful. Implementation of new technology at this time has added to pandemic stress levels greatly.
>
> *Nurse, intensive care, female, age 51–64*

> Why introduce a complete organisational change in work practice whilst the pandemic is in full flight? The increased stress and anxiety this causes is enormous.
>
> *Nurse, surgical, female, age 51–64*

A few healthcare workers spoke about pockets of resistance to change, which placed others at risk.

> We knew early on how infectious the virus was, but the arrogance of infection control services to insist on business-as-usual infection control is truly staggering.
>
> *Senior doctor, respiratory medicine, male, age 31–40*

> The main challenge is dealing with non-clinical staff who are very resistant to change, as they have worked in the practice for years. We had to make structural changes to the reception area on the weekend, as they would not agree to any changes. When I recommended to the owner that the reception staff should do a basic infection control course, I was told it was not necessary. It's so frustrating every day at work.
>
> *Nurse, general practice, female, age 51–64*

Other healthcare workers expressed a sense of loss, that the changes had taken away valued aspects of their role.

> Supporting staff to vent about missing aspects of our usual role is important. At the moment there are many of us who are doing a role that is very different to what it was pre-pandemic and we have all rolled with the punches to get the job done. The duration of the response is proving more fatiguing.
>
> *Occupational therapist, medical specialty, female, age 31–40*

> I suspect the change in work patterns may have altered healthcare workers' perceptions of work. It isn't even the COVID patients necessarily; the change in patient demographics in non-COVID patients has decreased work satisfaction levels. Less straightforward surgical patients with good outcomes, and an increased percentage of poor outcome patients—due to a reduction in surgical admissions in the ICU—has in my view led to healthcare worker fatigue, exhaustion, and potentially reduced longevity in their current roles.
>
> *Nurse, intensive care, male, age 51–64*

Redeployment

During the pandemic, some staff were redeployed into new roles. Some healthcare workers took this in their stride.

> Having to move from my normal job and having to work at multiple sites has been challenging but generally manageable. I'm glad to still be working.
>
> *Social worker, hospital aged care, female, age 51–64*

Many others found it stressful to be separated from their usual team and area of work.

> My main stressor during this period was working in a department where other junior medical staff had been redeployed, and I struggled working alone on a still reasonably busy ward. This coincided with the rollout of the electronic medical record, which I think made for quite a stressful period for the interns.
>
> *Junior doctor, respiratory medicine, female, age 20–30*

> Change of workflow and splitting of work teams can be uncomfortable.
>
> *Clinical scientist, pathology, female, age 51–64*

> Private health organisations need to stop forcing staff into redeployment, and leaving their own facilities short-staffed, which increases risk to staff and patients in these facilities.
>
> *Nurse, perioperative care, female, age 51–64*

> I specialise in a field and my ward has changed specialties so none of us are trained for the new patient population. It makes zero sense. Now the patients we would be taking care of are being cared for by less qualified nurses and we're not being utilised. It's moronic.
>
> *Nurse, medical specialty, male, age 31–40*

> Non-COVID wards were doing work that they wouldn't normally do or being redeployed as required. That strain is not something that is widely acknowledged.
>
> *Nurse, perioperative care, male, age 41–50*

> Our unit was uprooted with only a few days to move out. I personally had four days to pack up my office of twenty years. I am one of twelve staff whose workspace is still in limbo—working from home while our office is co-opted. This is very stressful.
>
> *Nurse, respiratory medicine, female, age 51–64*

Burnout

The outcome of overwork, staff shortages, and change described by healthcare workers was exhaustion and burnout. Many wrote about feeling physically and emotionally drained by the relentlessness of their work.

> COVID-19 has highlighted how burnt-out junior doctors are at baseline. The pandemic has added considerable stress to an already stressful roster for many. Acknowledgement from seniors of the hours we work and the risk we face would be a nice starting point.
>
> *Junior doctor, general medicine, female, age 20–30*

> It has been a very hard year physically and emotionally. I feel incredibly burnt out from not having a break from work.
>
> *Nurse, medical specialty, female, age 20–30*

> It's been a trying and challenging marathon period.
>
> *Nurse, surgical, female, age 51–64*

> I'm finding my job really draining and exhausting and more stressful than I can recall it ever being in 25 years of working as a doctor. It's been brutal.
>
> *General practitioner, female, age 51–64*

> I have found it to be very tiring, constantly wondering what has changed at work, and wondering if and when an outbreak will happen.
>
> *Nurse, medical specialty, female, age 41–50*

The ongoing pandemic has depleted my (and my colleagues') reserves. The hypervigilance has resulted in fatigue and with no relief at home this has been very draining.

Occupational therapist, medical specialty, female, age 41–50

It's been a huge year. We're all emotionally exhausted.

Nurse, surgical, female, age 20–30

It's been much more challenging than I ever expected it would be. I'm not sure if there's anything that would actually make our role any easier though. I feel like I'm emotionally exhausted from the months we've been dealing with the pressures of the entire situation, as has society in general.

Nurse, hospital aged care, female, age 51–64

Everyone is tired and run down. Thinking of now leaping into an elective surgery blitz is just exhausting.

Pharmacist, female, age 31–40

Being hyper-vigilant for extended periods of time is very tiring.

Speech pathologist, hospital aged care, female, age 41–50

I can't even begin to explain the extra physical and emotional burden that I've carried ever since COVID.

Nurse, female, age 20–30

Pre-existing burnout feelings have been significantly increased by the pandemic and I have no real idea how to change my situation.

Senior doctor, medical specialty, female, age 41–50

I think the fact that my summer holiday was cancelled due to bushfires, then COVID, has contributed to my burnout.

General practitioner, female, age 51–64

Sometimes I feel this is extremely draining, even though I'm seeing far less patients. Because many of these patients are complex, with multiple health complaints, I am less likely to have a profound impact on their quality of life or overall health. I've become very aware of this, and it's taxing mentally. At the moment, while there are "little wins", it feels like all "losses" and no "wins" which can burn you out.

Physiotherapist, community care, male, age 20–30

At the peak I regularly found myself thinking "I just can't anymore". But I did, and I guess I will keep on going. Now the caseload has dropped right

> back, and I feel as though I have been hit by a truck. If there's a third wave, I honestly don't think I would cope.
>
> *Nurse, hospital aged care, female, age 51–64*

> I'm burnt out. It's been really fucking hard.
>
> *Junior doctor, medical specialty, female, age 20–30*

Resignation

Some healthcare workers expressed their desire or need to leave their professions or organisations, either temporarily or permanently. They wrote about feeling drained of enthusiasm for jobs they once loved.

> It's been an awful time to work as a nurse and I have never hated it like this.
>
> *Nurse, general medicine, female, age 20–30*

> We joined a career we were proud of, we never thought it would mean putting those we love at risk; and getting so little back. I know colleagues, friends, who seriously regret being in healthcare now because they feel as though they are just being used, seen as a number and no more. The emotional toll of this pandemic on healthcare workers should not be taken lightly.
>
> *Nurse, emergency department, female, age 20–30*

> Almost every day I think about how much I don't want to be a nurse and how life would be easier in so many other jobs without the added stressors of shift work, sleep/wake cycle, high stakes, and rude people.
>
> *Nurse, emergency department, female, age 20–30*

> The cumulative stress is more than I think people realise, and that is why we are seeing so many staff leaving, or having to take extended leave, because they have hit the wall at the six-to-nine-month mark. This is a marathon—not a sprint—and most of us are not elite athletes with the psychology that goes with it.
>
> *Senior doctor, palliative care, female, age 41–50*

> I have seen so many frontline workers collapse emotionally and be treated that bad they leave.
>
> *Paramedic, male, age 41–50*

Some considered early retirement.

> If I could afford to, I would retire.
>
> *Nurse, surgical, female, age 51–64*

> It has brought forward my plans to retire from residential aged care.
>
> *Nurse, residential aged care, male, age 51–64*

> It has accelerated my planning for retirement from five years to within 12 months.
>
> *Senior doctor, medical specialty, male, age 51–64*

Many others told us they were considering a career change.

> Working directly with COVID patients. Witnessing your colleagues working so, so hard, with 12 hour shifts in an isolated room, struggling with ECMOs [extracorporeal membrane oxygenation]. This has taken a huge emotional toll on me, especially lately. To go from seeing what I see and do in the hospital, to then the social media world or news, and hearing community opinions that just have no idea. That breaks my heart and soul and I'm so, so tired. It makes me want to quit.
>
> *Nurse, intensive care, female, age 20–30*

> It's the first time in my career that I'm exhausted, lacking motivation and unable to cope with more change. It's challenging supporting junior staff. I'm seeking a career change as I feel burnt out and fatigued.
>
> *Nurse, community care, female, age 41–50*

> I have realised I no longer want to nurse and look forward to the day when I no longer have to. I look forward to what [comes] next for me, that is not as a nurse.
>
> *Nurse, medical specialty, female, age 41–50*

> I tested positive and was hotel quarantined for an extended period. It was the first time I needed to speak to a mental health professional. I love my profession, I am good at my profession, but the accumulated impact of COVID-19 has made me question whether it is worth it to continue sacrificing my own mental and physical health to look after the health of others.
>
> *Nurse, surgical, female, age 20–30*

> Being a junior doctor is hard enough. The pandemic has made me want to quit medicine even after spending most of my life striving towards being a doctor. I'm having a really hard time.
>
> *Junior doctor, general medicine, female, age 20–30*

> Personally, this year has made me rethink my career choices.
>
> *Junior doctor, intensive care, male, age 20–30*

> The pandemic has certainly made me reflect on my priorities and question my commitment to medicine.
>
> *General practitioner, female, age 41–50*

> I don't feel valued as a specialty trainee registrar. The pandemic has affected my outlook so much that I even imagine pursing an alternate career. I feel like the hospital is offering supports to look good or appear supportive, but actually they aren't. If they were supportive, they would help with rostering or more senior staff would help with workload. It just feels like we are sacrificing ourselves without any compensation and to be told we signed up for this is unhelpful. Our lives matter too.
>
> *Junior doctor, medical specialty, female, age 20–30*

> I'm just really tired. Lack of government backing of healthcare workers and adequate response with PPE or hospital systems to prevent spread within hospitals makes me often consider giving up work for quite a long time.
>
> *General practitioner, female, age 41–50*

> There is very little support for clinicians in private practice at high risk. I might resign and change careers.
>
> *General practitioner, female, age 41–50*

> The government response to COVID-19 and the impacts on my workplace have taken away most of the enjoyment of my work and I no longer look forward to coming to work. I have never felt like this before. I am considering how and when I will leave this job and that makes me sad.
>
> *Paramedic, male, age 41–50*

> After this pandemic is under control, I will be looking for a new position.
>
> *Nurse, medical specialty, female, age 31–40*

> Sadly, I think this pandemic will be career ending for some of the nurses in Victoria. Especially when having to be with dying patients everyday who could not have family or loved ones present.
>
> *Nurse, COVID clinic, female, age 41–50*

> It makes me want to give up medicine.
>
> *General practitioner, female, age 51–64*

Some had already taken active steps to move out of their current role.

> I am leaving ward-based work as a result of the pandemic. I find it unsustainable to keep doing shift work in this environment. I am moving to a research role.
>
> *Nurse, medical specialty, female, age 31–40*

I have looked for work outside of the ICU and am moving to a non-clinical role. The ICU is not a good place to work when you have a young family. I felt like a number and that my personal wellbeing was of little importance.

Nurse, intensive care, female, age 31–40

I was compelled to end up resigning due to dissatisfaction from not being heard and being drained from fighting for the safety of all my colleagues and for myself.

Nurse, intensive care, female, age 51–64

When our department has been under stress and higher workloads, they didn't do anything to staff up or offer us extra supports. If anything, we were told we needed to step up further. We were already giving 110 percent. Ultimately, they do not care at all for frontline workers. Hence why after working for the same organisation for 18 years and the last 12 in a public emergency department, I have resigned. My workplace response to their workers during COVID-19 is the reason for my resignation.

Nurse, emergency department, female, age 41–50

COVID-19 has honestly made me want to change jobs and leave nursing. I'm currently waiting to hear if I am successful in gaining entrance to a new course in 2021. Working on a COVID ward exposing myself and family to a very infectious virus with no hazard pay is the straw that broke the camel's back!

Nurse, general medicine, female, age 41–50

I am actually about to resign and relocate interstate because it just too much!

Allied health practitioner, emergency department, female, age 20–30

I've applied for work interstate in February—Victoria going it alone is just miserable.

Junior doctor, emergency department, female, age 31–40

I have left the pharmacy profession due to the COVID pandemic, due to horrific behaviour from patients and lack of support and recognition.

Pharmacist, community care, female, age 20–30

9

LEADERSHIP AND TEAMS

> I felt safe and supported by the strategies implemented by the Nurse Unit Manager in my ward who has been an exceptional leader (leading by example). I also felt that I was able to strongly adapt to the positive changes made in my ward due to the support of the excellent team that I work with.
>
> *Nurse, general medicine, female, age 31–40*

The COVID-19 pandemic functioned as a kind of truth serum, revealing the effectiveness of leaders and the culture of teams, with little ability to hide behind rhetoric or platitudes. This chapter discusses the qualities of effective and ineffective leaders, and the characteristics of healthy and unhealthy teams, as perceived by frontline healthcare workers. Healthcare workers described how some people in formal positions of authority were ineffective leaders, while others with no official leadership title or role shone in their ability to inspire and unite those around them. At a time when people were disconnected from other supports and structures, the culture of teams took on new significance. For some, colleagues became as close as family, the only people who really understood what they were going through. Other health workers found themselves trapped in an unpleasant working environment with little team support.

Leaders

At a global level, the pandemic revealed vast chasms between different leadership styles, reflected in the effectiveness of countries' pandemic responses and care for the most vulnerable members of communities. Healthcare workers also wrote about their diverse experiences of leadership.

Some expressed gratitude and respect for leaders at a team, organisational, and governmental level.

DOI: 10.4324/9781003228394-9

Great leadership from the top down helped things to run smoothly despite all the changes.

Junior doctor, emergency department, male, age 31–40

The current "kindness" pandemic has been applied well within our hospital's culture and communication has overall been excellent. Interdepartmental support/training has never been better—hope all these things continue and become permanent. Staff feel valued and safe and perform better with these attitudes from all levels of management, clinical and non-clinical.

Junior doctor, emergency department, female, age 51–64

Managerial level feedback acknowledging day-to-day challenges posed by COVID has been beneficial in boosting morale. My Nurse Unit Manager's ability to maintain a steady supply of PPE has been incredibly helpful.

Nurse, emergency department, male, age 31–40

I work in a great place with wonderful leaders who have done an exemplary job in preparing and implementing all the planning.

Nurse, intensive care, female, age 51–64

Our ICU, especially the management team, were incredible. Their preparation and support ensured staff were confident in our ability to get the job done.

Nurse, intensive care, female, age 41–50

Thank you to management for all they have done to keep us all sane and safe.

Administrative worker, respiratory medicine, female, age 41–50

I thank the politicians, Chief Medical Officers, and Chief Health Officers for their extraordinary commitment and very strong leadership. I feel they have our back, and we are in this together for the community.

Senior doctor, medical specialty, male, age 51–64

Others were scathing about the role of some managers and politicians in responding to the crisis.

Leadership at several levels has let the state of Victoria down. This is readily reflected by hospital management: they are removed, any efforts at engagement are superficial, no clinical involvement gives them no credibility. This feeling has not evolved overnight—over the years there has been an ongoing disconnect with a palpable disregard festering on the part of management—e.g., unrealistic KPIs are obstacles to good care, electronic medical record inadequacy. The good thing about crises is that when (or if) they end all actors will emerge with the reputations they deserve.

Senior doctor, emergency department, male, age 51–64

> Lack of support from my employer left me feeling alone and abandoned. If you make a mistake, you're chastised and made an example of in front of others, belittled, left feeling worthless.
>
> *Paramedic, male, age 41–50*

> Unity of political leadership through the pandemic is crucial. Political point-scoring by the federal government in the second wave has been counterproductive, and frankly disgusting.
>
> *Junior doctor, general medicine, male, age 31–40*

> My workplace has a reformatory management style where management treat us all with suspicion, and assume we are all doing—or are going to do—the "wrong thing" and must be carefully watched.
>
> *Social worker, community care, female, age 51–64*

> Even though it has not truly affected me, the fear of the possible is very difficult and scary. I feel very unsupported by the heads of my department; they send out very format type emails that really don't mean anything! We are in this on our own!
>
> *Senior doctor, general medicine, male, age 51–64*

> The problems … stem from a deliberate policy of excluding experienced healthcare workers from key decision-making. They actively denigrate doctors in private meetings and have several layers of bureaucrats between the Minister and the Chief Health Officer.
>
> *Senior doctor, emergency department, male, age 51–64*

> Criticism from [Australian Prime Minister] Scott Morrison regarding how the state of Victoria is dealing with COVID-19 is not appreciated and most unhelpful as we are all doing our best and doing it tough.
>
> *Nurse, intensive care, male, age 51–64*

The need for evidence-informed leadership decisions

Many healthcare workers voiced concern about what they regarded as lack of evidence-based decisions. As discussed in Chapter 7, they wanted leaders to prioritise safety at work, and to pay attention to emerging evidence in formulating and updating guidelines. A particular example was emerging evidence about aerosol transmission.

> The whole argument that there was "no evidence" of aerosol spread—and therefore higher levels of PPE were not required—was misguided. It would have been much easier to control the anxiety of healthcare workers if the message had been: "There is no evidence of aerosol spread, but there is also

no evidence that it is not being spread by aerosol. We value our staff and will provide the highest level of protection until the evidence proves that this is not required."

Senior doctor, intensive care, male, age 41–50

I have concerns about new science around transmission being dismissed. It's very stressful to have the Infection Control Expert Group making recommendations on infection control, and just assuming the transmission is the same as "traditional respiratory viral transmission" which they don't really understand anyway, especially aerosol science.

Senior doctor, emergency department, male, age 51–64

I feel that some decisions made at a higher level were not based on good evidence, such as the ban on water births, due to a lack of knowledge on facilitating this form of care from policy makers.

Midwife, female, age 51–64

The qualities of good leadership

Healthcare workers were clear about what they were looking for, or had experienced, in a good leader: someone with their feet on the ground, their ears open to hearing from frontline staff and experts, the backbone to take decisive action when needed, and their heart in the right place.

We need more attunement from management and government to the actual realities of care provision on the ground.

Senior doctor, medical specialty, male, age 31–40

Kind but strong leadership that is visible and around the wards.

Senior doctor, medical specialty, female, age 65–70

The support of senior nursing staff was appreciated. They would come by and give the thumbs up signal through the glass.

Nurse, intensive care, female, age 51–64

Having the support of good managers and a friendly team has been invaluable. Fortunately, we, as a team, are given the opportunity to speak openly and frankly during our pre-shift huddles. Issues raised are generally dealt with in a timely manner.

Nurse, community care, female, age 51–64

The response by the leadership in our anaesthetic department was outstanding. We have had quite a few trainees who have come from other hospitals who were very happy to be working here. It was great to see that our department

> values its staff by the PPE, the training, the simulations, the interface with other departments, and the COVID intubating teams.
>
> *Senior doctor, anaesthetics, female, age 41–50*

> Having strong leadership and management in the hospital is very important.
>
> *Junior doctor, surgical, female, age 31–40*

> Knowing that we have support from our managers, seeing them help on the floor and talking to us all the time … I liked the way my hospital acted very quickly in their decisions for staff and patient safety.
>
> *Nurse, general medicine, female, age 20–30*

> Knowing that you are supported by management and encouraged to correctly use proper PPE is important. Feeling that you are being taken care of.
>
> *Nurse, intensive care, male, age 41–50*

> Proactive, ethical bosses make the biggest difference.
>
> *Pharmacist, female, age 20–30*

When good leadership is absent or invisible

Some leaders were not visible on the frontline of care, were perceived as not caring about their staff, and focused on bureaucratic indicators rather than providing the leadership needed during this time.

> We continually get emails telling us what we can't do and what we must do, but NEVER have we had a visit to acknowledge the daily stress we have of delivering a face-to-face service to the community.
>
> *Nurse, community care, female, age 51–64*

> A show of compassion by management and a real presence by them. I can't remember what they look like.
>
> *Nurse, emergency department, female, age 51–64*

> At a time where tangible leadership was needed the executive were working from home (as directed by the Health Department), visible mostly by Zoom leaving staff to implement the management directives as best they could—so leadership on the ground is needed. I never saw any member of the executive/management in full PPE in this entire time.
>
> *Senior doctor, surgical, female, age 51–64*

> People who claim to be "frontline", but are actually not clinical, spouting how things should be done and how us—on the actual patient care side of things—should be conducting ourselves. Consultants [senior doctors] were

> particularly obnoxious—they hid in their offices and sent out WhatsApp messages on how to suck eggs without having the balls to come bedside. Idiotic directives from our upper management working from home were on about the same level.
>
> *Nurse, intensive care, female, age 41–50*

> Executives are safe in their nice office, or working from home with big pay checks, not dealing face-to-face with patients daily. They're out of touch.
>
> *Administrative worker, surgical, female, age 20–30*

> Management must support staff in-person, not hide away in their ivory towers … I realise that this is something none of us have ever lived through before and people are trying but some managers are finding it easier to hide away and protect themselves.
>
> *Nurse, medical specialty, female, age 51–64*

> I was disappointed that senior management was nowhere to be seen at the height and even today they are not visible. Email communication is important but being visible and talking to staff is also essential to get the best out of staff.
>
> *Nurse, surgical, female, age 41–50*

Some healthcare workers in frontline roles were critical of hospital administrators for slow decision-making and not providing timely guidance to staff. They described needing to step up to fill a void left by those in formal positions of authority.

> One big thing that I have learned during this time is that we have to get on with it and make decisions for ourselves and our teams rather than waiting for the executives to reach any decision. If I had waited for appropriate advice, I may well have had an entire team furloughed or burned out from the stress.
>
> *Senior doctor, palliative care, female, age 51–64*

Healthcare workers wanted governmental and organisational leaders who were cohesive and coordinated in their approach, decisive, took actions, and were responsive to their needs.

> Too many hospital executives and Department of Health leaders showed a reluctance to act.
>
> *Senior doctor, general medicine, male, age 41–50*

> On the ground decision-making is slow, and often I never get a response to queries. The response has to go through so many levels of management for an answer, that the query gets lost in the ether.
>
> *Occupational therapist, community care, female, age 51–64*

> The ability of management to implement rapid and responsive change is essential. Pondering over, or asking to "take time to consider", changes led to unnecessary stress for staff on the front line.
>
> *Respiratory scientist, female, age 51–64*

> While emotional support during a crisis is critical, it won't help me if I end up in ICU because the government failed to take the minimum standards required to keep me safe. I don't want an apology after the fact, I want action taken now to prevent the morbidity and mortality of healthcare workers.
>
> *Junior doctor, anaesthetics, female, age 31–40*

> I have worked in a very proactive department. However, I have constantly felt let down by the executive and governmental response. The safety of my co-workers and management of the pandemic has been achieved through individual efforts on the local scale, and I am thoroughly disappointed with the lack of a coordinated response at a regional, state and federal level.
>
> *General practitioner, female, age 51–64*

> The government and community leaders can do more to help us deal with a sense of impending doom which is much worse when there is lack of cohesive leadership.
>
> *Senior doctor, medical specialty, female, age 31–40*

They also wanted leaders who understood what the problems were "on the ground" rather than making assumptions about what the challenges were.

> There was a disconnect between "frontline issues" and what the executive told us the problems were.
>
> *Senior doctor, emergency department, male, age 51–64*

> It's not great when you have non-clinical people making clinical decisions that affect you, but they have no experience of being on a ward and the logistics of managing patients in Level Four PPE [the highest level of protection].
>
> *Physiotherapist, surgical, female, age 20–30*

The challenges of being a leader

Those who were themselves in leadership roles spoke candidly about the challenges they faced.

> At an executive level, the workload has been relentless, and it's been very difficult managing the expectation of other executives and the Board to

> continue our day jobs, whilst dealing with so many new things that we have no frame of reference for.
>
> *Leader, female, age 31–40*

> It can be quite isolating being in a management role, having to implement things that may not be popular with staff, families, and residents in aged care.
>
> *Nurse, residential aged care, female, age 51–64*

> I have found it difficult as a manager to deal with a number of complaints and negative remarks about policies implemented as a result of COVID. It seems a hard task to keep everyone happy during this time despite best efforts.
>
> *Nurse, palliative care, female, age 31–40*

These challenges spanned having to rapidly make decisions—in a relentlessly changing environment with no established frame of reference— to feeling isolated and lacking supports.

> As a nursing team leader, I am constantly making decisions that I have little to no experience for, that impact on my patients, the team I lead, and could potentially have dire impacts on my community. I feel isolated from my usual supports as their COVID-19 experiences are so different and I feel limited with how much I can share … I know I am anxious, but actually there is good reason for my anxiety. And if I don't keep doing what I do there is no back up plan, as so many of my team have been redeployed.
>
> *Nurse, respiratory medicine, female, age 51–64*

> The impact of rapidly presented new information, and changing how we work, cannot be underestimated. It is exhausting and difficult and time-consuming to communicate with your team.
>
> *Nurse, general medicine, female, age 41–50*

> I hark back to the uncertainty, the ever-changing situation. I coined a title to describe how I felt during many weeks of the pandemic "COVID PTSD". I would sit in my office fielding phone calls and emails, answering constant questions, and educating staff. Dealing with issues about things constantly changing. I found that when there was a pause in the flood of phone calls etc., I would not be able to settle into doing any of my regular infection control work. I would sit at my desk, on edge, waiting for the phone to ring again, unable to stop my anxiety from climbing. It has been exhausting. Coupled with lying awake at night worrying about whether I had done everything I possibly could. Was I doing my job properly and efficiently? Was I protecting the staff well enough? It has been a very trying time.
>
> *Senior doctor, infectious diseases, female, age 51–64*

The pandemic increased the workload of those in leadership roles with no commensurate increase in resources.

> As a Nurse Unit Manager, I work over 50 hours a week and feel utter tiredness and sadness. I am burnt out. How can I run a team while I am constantly putting out "spot fires"? I don't even get paid for the time required to do my role.
>
> *Nurse, surgical, female, age 41–50*

> We need recognition from senior management that middle managers' jobs were too big prior to the pandemic. The extra unpaid work associated with the pandemic needs more recognition. I've worked up to 20 hours extra most weeks unpaid.
>
> *Occupational therapist, community care, female, age 51–64*

Some felt thrust into leadership roles or positions of increased responsibility without warning or support.

> I was rung five minutes before shift started and told "you are being moved to a new aged care ward and you are in charge". Even though I had never worked there, and only had agency junior staff to work with in hot [COVID-19] areas.
>
> *Nurse, hospital aged care, female, age 51–64*

> I can see the strain on my consultants [senior doctors] and feel I have an increased responsibility to function at a level above my senior registrar position, and increased responsibilities to support more junior medical staff and nursing and allied health staff.
>
> *Junior doctor, palliative care, male, age 41–50*

Many clinical leaders expressed a deep sense of care for their staff and concern for their wellbeing, and complex feelings of guilt and distress when unable to provide them with adequate protection.

> Holding the fear and anger of all my staff, while managing my own fears for their safety. Fears that we would be unable to provide basic care to people. Fear of finishing it all with PTSD. Long hours and constant change.
>
> *Senior doctor, emergency department, male, age 41–50*

> I was coping well and supporting my staff well until I was asked to do something which was right against what I would normally do, and was too great a challenge for me to do, as I felt it was against the best interests of my staff and my unit. This caused me to become very stressed and tearful for some weeks … I value my staff and the very dedicated team I work with.
>
> *Nurse, general medicine, female, age 65–70*

> Owning a practice, rapidly changing the business in a physical sense and business sense and how we practiced medicine. It changed overnight to keep everyone as safe as possible … I had many sleepless nights worrying about everyone's safety and keeping the business going.
>
> *General practitioner, female, age 51–64*

> As a Clinical Director of an emergency department, there have also been worries of responsibility for my staff working on the frontline.
>
> *Senior doctor, emergency department, female, age 41–50*

> Administrative colleagues are hugely stressed, and guilt-ridden after following guidelines which are shown to be wrong.
>
> *Senior doctor, general medicine, male, age 65–70*

> I had a feeling of being a powerless "middleman" between frontline clinical staff—who were calling for increased PPE—and higher hospital management who refused to entertain any dissenting opinions.
>
> *Senior doctor, anaesthetics, male, age 41–50*

They also identified the lack of supports for those in management and leadership roles.

> We're being expected to deliver on business as usual, in addition to significant additional responsibilities, with no additional resources.
>
> *Leader, infectious diseases, female, age 51–64*

> There has been a large focus on maintaining wellbeing for carers and nurses, but management have had more negative recognition. Managing an aged care facility is extremely difficult and I think facility managers and care managers deserve more support.
>
> *Nurse, residential aged care, female, age 20–30*

> Leaders are not being supported enough: they're giving all the time and need peers to check in on them.
>
> *Orthoptist, female, age 51–64*

Teams

Across all kinds of roles and responsibilities, workplace colleagues were identified as a crucial support during the pandemic.

> You need a good team environment to be able to cope with the extra challenges and difficulties caused by pandemic.
>
> *Clinical scientist, medical specialty, female, age 51–64*

> Great colleagues make for a great workplace environment, which makes for better mental health for staff and better care for patients!
>
> *Nurse, emergency department, female, age 41–50*

> Working in a close-knit team gives you both professional and moral support.
>
> *Nurse, emergency department, female, age 51–64*

> Having a supportive and welcoming staff environment on my current ward has made such a huge difference and helped me still want to come to work or not get too bogged down about COVID while on shift.
>
> *Nurse, medical specialty, female, age 20–30*

> The most useful and practical support I've found is good colleagues, a supportive workplace, and coffee.
>
> *Nurse, community care, female, age 31–40*

Strengthening teams and working together

Some healthcare workers felt that the pandemic had brought their teams closer together.

> I am constantly in awe of the work that my colleagues are doing. We have banded together to look after each other at work.
>
> *Nurse, emergency department, female, age 31–40*

> It has united healthcare in never-before-seen ways. It has taken the "competition" out of the system. All doctors, everywhere, want the same things and want to work together. The increase in camaraderie between nurses is fantastic.
>
> *Nurse, intensive care, female, age 20–30*

> I feel much more connected to my co-workers having gone through this experience together.
>
> *Nurse, intensive care, female, age 20–30*

> The relationships in my immediate work environment have been strengthened during the pandemic. Being included in discussions and watching the anaesthetists work together to solve problems and plan was very comforting during the most stressful times of the pandemic. Being part of a cohesive team helped enormously … My own team's response kept me going every day.
>
> *Nurse, surgical, female, age 41–50*

> I am lucky to work in a great department, led by good people and with amazing colleagues who I now count as friends. I have been here not quite

a year and I cannot imagine working anywhere else. My last two workplaces were awful, and I am so glad I am not trying to deal with this there.

Radiographer, medical imaging, female, age 31–40

We've been fortunate to have compassionate leadership in the hospital I've been redeployed to. In my usual workplace, what was less than helpful there, was commentary about us being lucky to have a job—not helpful when you are experiencing fear. So, it was really nice when redeployed to be hearing acknowledgement of feelings of fear and concern for personal and family wellbeing. Really good sense of team in the hospital I've been redeployed too.

Nurse, perioperative care, female, age 51–64

I feel that intensive care at my hospital have been doing a fantastic job. From the cleaners, administrative workers, right through to the nurses and doctors, we are a team and have displayed that time and time again.

Administrative worker, intensive care, female, age 51–64

The nurses and team that I have interacted with are pretty much all kind, welcoming, patient folks who really put the patients first. We are so lucky to have a team like that, and I am so lucky to be a part of it.

Administrative worker, emergency department, female, age 31–40

The pandemic has bound together our department. It has also meant fabulous collaborations around the hospital. It has caused me to lift in my role and really develop my leadership. In many ways it has been a wonderful thing to be a part of and—given that it had to happen—I'm glad to have had this chance to serve the community at such an important time. But I'm tired and I'm sad and I miss the joyful life I led before it came.

Senior doctor, emergency department, male, age 41–50

I have worked in aged care with COVID-positive patients, some who have died and others who have survived. It is really hard to explain what this work is like to others who haven't experienced it. It's so different from any other work I have done. The only people that can really support me are those who have been through it too—we have become a tight little group, separated from our other colleagues. PTSD is a real concern for many.

Nurse, hospital aged care, female, age 41–50

Teams that thrived during the pandemic made it a priority to stay connected despite the restrictions.

Connecting outside of core work activity is important.

Administrative worker, female, age 31–40

> Doing things that maintain a sense of team, like social events with work colleagues, is helpful.
>
> *Physiotherapist, intensive care, female, age 31–40*

> Our department has made a very conscious effort to keep everyone connected from afar—creation of WebEx teams for daily memes and happy stories, daily sing-a-longs via WebEx, we had a department trivia night.
>
> *Physiotherapist, respiratory medicine, female, age 31–40*

> We have a catch-up session in aged care weekly on Zoom. Although it does not provide specific strategies for stress/anxiety, the camaraderie between colleagues is reassuring.
>
> *Junior doctor, medical specialty, female, age 20–30*

Healthcare workers valued team cultures which were caring and where team members looked out for each other.

> I think that it's useful to keep an eye out for your co-workers, ask them if they're OK, encourage them to take a break if they're showing signs of burnout. The trouble is that it's more difficult in the current setting: with social distancing you may not run into colleagues in the usual meeting spots and communication is less reliable across group videoconferences or with masks in place.
>
> *Senior doctor, respiratory medicine, female, age 51–64*

> Good communication from the Department of Health. It has made being vulnerable OK, and this has changed the dynamic in our team for the better.
>
> *Nurse, community care, female, age 51–64*

> Checking in with colleagues to make sure they are doing well helps immensely in both keeping everyone content but also helping us grow closer as people.
>
> *Administrative worker, medical imaging, male, age 20–30*

Healthcare workers described benefits of being able to debrief with colleagues.

> Debriefing at the end of each shift is a positive thing to do.
>
> *General practitioner, male, age 41–50*

> Being able to talk to my peers is a big help with managing my feelings regarding this pandemic.
>
> *Nurse, intensive care, female, age 20–30*

> Supportive colleagues who understand are an amazing blessing.
>
> *Senior doctor, respiratory medicine, female, age 41–50*

> My team at work are similarly-minded people. I found them helpful to talk to.
>
> *Nurse, community care, female, age 41–50*

> The value of grabbing a coffee at the end of the ward round, and taking time out for 10 minutes as a team, is very important.
>
> *Senior doctor, surgical, female, age 41–50*

> Being able to decompress with colleagues is vital. At times it has been difficult to find somewhere a group of us can sit together due to restrictions on numbers in the one room, but as the weather warms up, we have been able to sit out in our garden which is lovely.
>
> *Nurse, community care, female, age 31–40*

Healthcare workers also drew on the wisdom of healthcare workers around the world in preparing for, and adapting to, new challenges.

> Networking with other health care professionals around the world to share and learn from their experience.
>
> *General practitioner, female, age 41–50*

> For me it's been really useful to share ideas and experiences with ICU staff from the UK, US, and Canada via social media. Building greater camaraderie amongst our staff has also helped a lot.
>
> *Nurse, intensive care, female, age 41–50*

The dynamics of disconnected teams

Not all healthcare workers described such positive experiences within their teams during the pandemic. Some wrote about feeling disconnected from their colleagues due to changed work conditions, including public health restrictions on face-to-face meetings, and the loss of spontaneous corridor conversations.

> One of the things though that has always made work easier is just being together or having unit meetings and little debriefs in the corridor which aren't really possible at the moment. Changing from a telephone conference unit meeting to a WebEx where we could see each other made a difference to morale.
>
> *Senior doctor, general medicine, female, age 41–50*

> Our collegiality, and ability to share knowledge, has been severely compromised by the changes in the way we work.
>
> *Senior doctor, general medicine, male, age 41–50*

> Sometimes all we want is to hear someone say "thank you" or ask you how you are. It's a simple thing that will brighten your day. Being in a team that lacks communication is a big challenge and struggle. There's no small talk or "chit chat".
>
> *Administrative worker, medical imaging, female, age 20–30*

> Being so separated from my peers has had a massive impact on my wellbeing.
>
> *Nurse, surgical, female, age 20–30*

> We barely have any time together except for work on the floor. I don't know who is on shift half the time, because now we leave to go on the floor as soon as our names are ticked off.
>
> *Nurse, emergency department, female, age 20–30*

> Right now, in my work environment, we actually don't have a direct manager that is looking out for us. Other areas … have 2–3 weekly huddles to touch base to see how everyone is going, so that makes me feel secluded, and also exacerbates the fact that I am single and live alone. I have no one at work nor home to see if I am OK. I have a few colleagues who do a great job all touching base as do I for them … and I also try and do a walk a few times a week at lunchtimes with colleagues for some fresh air and exercise, but I just don't feel included or part of a team at all.
>
> *Nurse, female, age 31–40*

Healthcare workers spoke about the importance of tearooms as a place to connect and catch-up, and the role of shared food in celebrating occasions and connecting with colleagues. These opportunities were greatly missed.

> Removal of the ability to connect with colleagues in the workplace because of risk of tearoom contagion has removed a large part of my unofficial support network. We have no spaces available for brief catchups in a safe and socially distanced way.
>
> *Senior doctor, medical specialty, female, age 41–50*

> Worst of all, the tearoom at work has been taken away from us, forcing us to find elsewhere to eat, and the debrief with other work colleagues can no longer occur. There is no-one to debrief with about the difficulties and stress. The ward continues to work as usual but communication between Nurse Unit Manager, senior and junior nurses is non-existent. No ward meetings and no discussions, increases the feelings of isolation.
>
> *Nurse, emergency department, female, age 51–64*

> Separating for meal breaks, no drinks in the workspace, and no shared food on nights has been hard.
>
> *Nurse, emergency department, female, age 41–50*

> It has been hard to keep up social activities at work, such as birthday cakes and farewell functions, due to restrictions. This is having an ongoing impact. This is affecting work friendships and relationships and enjoyment of work.
>
> *Physiotherapist, medical specialty, female, age 51–64*

> I would love the opportunity to get dressed up and go out with fellow frontline workers to an event that celebrates our efforts to overcome this pandemic.
>
> *Nurse, community care, female, age 41–50*

Some healthcare workers lamented that the pandemic had accentuated negative workplace dynamics and brought out the worst in people.

> The pandemic has exacerbated negative workplace dynamics and highlighted bad leadership.
>
> *Senior doctor, emergency department, female, age 31–40*

> It's been eye-opening about humanity. It's brought out the worst in a lot of people. People you would expect to be more caring and supportive have not been that way at all.
>
> *Social worker, emergency department, female, age 41–50*

> In the workplace during the COVID-19 pandemic I have experienced: 1) bullying, isolation, and exclusion, 2) exploitation of good will and strong work ethic, and 3) being disregarded, disrespected, and invalidated in the health services I work in.
>
> *Physiotherapist, hospital outpatients, female, age 41–50*

> Frontline means caring for the patients. I found my unit was carried away with a lot of back patting and glory hunting from supernumerary and other staff that did not gear up and care at the bedside for any time, let alone 12 hours. A lot of covert narcissism went viral during this period, and I found if you were tough about demanding a rotation away from caring for COVID you were taken advantage of and thrown in. My unit did that to a number of good-natured nurses with less than five years' experience because it seemed they knew they could. As a result, one in particular is exhibiting strong symptoms of PTSD, and will not get help because no one will check-in and see how we're coping as individuals. We've been depersonalised to a workforce by this pandemic and for a time there it felt we were regarded as disposable as the poor bloody nursing home patients that became infected.
>
> *Nurse, intensive care, female, age 41–50*

> Disintegration and lack of respect between colleagues, amplified by social media, empire-building, career-building colleagues that sought to personally profit from the pandemic at the expense of others.
>
> *Senior doctor, infectious diseases, male, age 31–40*

> I've witnessed some awful human behaviour during this pandemic. I feel so many professionals have lost their humanity.
>
> *Nurse, hospital aged care, female, age 51–64*

A small number of healthcare workers had difficulty understanding, or empathising with, the emotional responses of team members to the stresses of the pandemic.

> I have found it much more difficult to deal with the significant anxieties of others than the pandemic. This has made the workplace very unpleasant and stressful. I think that the response of my hospital has been pretty good all things considered, but the intense emotional response from a small number of colleagues has made the atmosphere within the department almost unbearable.
>
> *Senior doctor, anaesthetics, female, age 41–50*

> I have been disappointed by some of the extreme anxiety and behavioural responses in a few clinical colleagues who appear lacking in resilience even though the actual direct impact on them has been negligible. Some of them withdrew from clinical aspects of work with little notice or rational reason and left others to take on additional work and responsibilities. It has left me questioning their suitability for their chosen professional roles. All other aspects of the COVID-related response have been generally very positive, and I have been really pleased with the collegiality, positive approach and support shared within my clinical team. Patient care and protection of staff have been the key elements of the response.
>
> *Senior doctor, intensive care, male, age 41–50*

Others felt that everyone was doing their best, but that fatigue was beginning to depress team morale.

> My work colleagues were excellent in the beginning and coped very well with the early adoption of new strategies, but the stress and burnout started to show after a few months of the COVID restrictions. Staff who were usually positive started to become more negative and unwilling to accept any more changes to their work. Morale at my workplace is the lowest it has ever been, and I work with a great bunch of dedicated, caring professionals.
>
> *Occupational therapist, community care, female, age 51–64*

10

COMMUNICATION AND UNDERSTANDING

> At all times good communication and transparency are important but this has been especially true at this time [during the pandemic] and the lack of it is so noticeable.
>
> *Allied health practitioner, rehabilitation, female, age 31–40*

Communication needs and strategies, digital approaches to care, and information seeking were hallmarks of being a healthcare worker during the pandemic. In this chapter we present the central communication and information challenges they faced. Healthcare workers told us that to do their jobs effectively, they needed transparent, timely, and consistent information. They also wanted to be in dialogue with their leaders—with their concerns heard and responded to. Communication at work changed profoundly in response to the pandemic, with the dramatic entrance of telehealth from the wings of healthcare to centre stage. Healthcare workers acknowledged the benefits of telehealth, but also told us about its challenges. Finally, healthcare workers talked about navigating both social and traditional media. While appreciating the value of social media in providing them with up-to-date information, and keeping them connected, they worried about sensationalist reporting and damaging posts in both social and traditional media.

Communication needs

Healthcare workers told us that clear communication was essential to their ability to manage their work and their fears. Accuracy of information was particularly important due to the amount of misinformation being shared during the pandemic.

DOI: 10.4324/9781003228394-10

> Information from up-line management is helpful. Knowing what is going on is better than worrying about vague plans or getting asked questions you can't answer.
>
> *Nurse, medical specialty, female, age 51–64*

> I think there is a lot of information out there that is useful but filtering out the rubbish is challenging at times.
>
> *Occupational therapist, hospital aged care, female, age 51–64*

> The Chief Health Officers of all the States have been in the forefront of providing excellent information. I have valued this.
>
> *General practitioner, female, age 71+*

> I've experienced two different communication styles between the private and public hospitals. Public hospital communication is fantastic: I receive daily statistics, the Nurse Unit Manager regularly checks in on staff, there is a WhatsApp group for rapid communication within the department, extensive and repeated training. In my private sector job: no communication, no statistics, positive cases not disclosed to staff.
>
> *Nurse, perioperative care, female, age 41–50*

The qualities of good communication

Healthcare workers told us that communication of information should be open and transparent, regular and timely, and as clear and consistent as possible.

> Support of our leadership team has been amazing, [we've] benefited from clear, concise, and open communication.
>
> *Nurse, emergency department, female, age 31–40*

> There needs to be an obligation for transparency of information from hospital directors to the public, and to staff, regarding COVID case numbers, actual risks, and gaps in processes. Staff feel unheard and disregarded and unnecessarily placed at risk.
>
> *Administrative worker, hospital aged care, female, age 41–50*

> An open communication channel with the leader is very important to institute changes and improvement in this crisis.
>
> *Senior doctor, surgical specialty, male, age 41–50*

> Good communication is the key. If you receive good communication, you are able to make good decisions and I try to always provide good and effective communication to my team.
>
> *Manager, general practice, female, age 41–50*

Conversely, healthcare workers described how perceptions of secrecy and withholding of information led to unnecessary anxiety.

> Management need to be more careful about not isolating staff and providing clear communication.
>
> *Nurse, medical specialty, male, age 51–64*

> It's annoying knowing things are being discussed, but waiting for the email, then having a finger pointed at you for not already doing something you were just informed about.
>
> *Dental practitioner, female, age 41–50*

> Hidden memos—that will affect us—were distributed to the executive but not to us. It was very frustrating.
>
> *Junior doctor, general medicine, female, age 31–40*

> We need transparency in the department. As a non-nurse, non-doctor we are often not privy to why things are happening.
>
> *Technician, emergency department, female, age 41–50*

Due to the rapid pace of change, information updates needed to be regular and timely.

> We need timely explanation of epidemiological data and disclosure of data and how certain decisions are made.
>
> *General practitioner, female, age 41–50*

> Get clear messages out in a timely manner.
>
> *Nurse, community care, female, age 65–70*

> Having real time data and numbers would be good. Feel like you do all the work, at a testing clinic, and not know the outcomes.
>
> *Nurse, community care, female, age 31–40*

> Frequent updates from management help.
>
> *Nurse, hospital aged care, female, age 41–50*

> Our unit was very positive in updating the staff on a regular basis. I found this much better than the overwhelming environment of the news and social media. We had a live update every few days from the Nurse Unit Manager about what is happening and what we are doing and what is changing re protocols.
>
> *Nurse, intensive care, female, age 20–30*

> I find the twice-weekly employee forums very useful and a great resource. They have made me feel very much part of the organisation and I have enjoyed the presentations immensely.
>
> *Nurse, hospital aged care, female, age 51–64*

> We need daily team meetings where ALL team members are kept up to date and have a forum to ask questions.
>
> *Nurse, hospital aged care, female, age 20–30*

Healthcare workers sought clear and consistent information to be able to do their jobs well.

> Clear, well-phrased directions are essential for safe communication in both restrictions and precautions.
>
> *Nurse, community care, female, age 41–50*

> I work in operating theatres, and I felt there was no clear advice on how to treat COVID patients in operating theatres.
>
> *Nurse, perioperative care, female, age 31–40*

> Clear consistent policies need to be in place without the possibility of individual interpretation to allow a united and consistent approach to everything from who gets tested, who tests, to how to support one another.
>
> *Senior doctor, palliative care, male, age 31–40*

> I am a community worker, but my partner is a manager of an allied health team in a hospital setting. The stress of both our workplaces and lack of communication and clear directives was incredibly stressful. I think that in times of crisis, leadership and management need to understand the power of providing support and validating experience: "Yep, this is just stressful." Allowing leave, checking in, etc. But they also need a presence and a clear attack of communication and action plans.
>
> *Occupational therapist, community care, female, age 31–40*

Receiving different advice from different sources was a common challenge.

> A single source of information for GPs would have helped.
>
> *General practitioner, female, age 51–64*

> Consistent messaging is really important. There's only so much you can read: do I defer to information from my workplaces, college, Ahpra [Australian Health Practitioner Regulation Agency], AMA [Australian Medical Association], my medical defence organisation, Health Pathways, special interest groups I'm

subscribed to … or others? Or do I attend yet another videoconference online? The amount of information is exhausting and keeping abreast of the changing clinical guidelines only adds to that.

General practitioner, female, age 31–40

Biggest issues are inconsistent approaches between hospitals and having to follow different protocols depending on where patients are transported. It's hard to know what we are doing at times as it changes so often, often mid-shift with no notification.

Paramedic, female, age 41–50

There needs to be better co-ordination of information and resources from government and primary care.

General practitioner, male, age 41–50

Healthcare workers told us they found it particularly frustrating when leaders said one thing, and then did another.

Management communication with guidelines needs to be clear and concise. You cannot tell people to maintain rules when you are continuously relaxing the rules at a whim, or if the manager finds it too difficult to enforce.

Administrative worker, hospital aged care, female, age 51–64

Our hospital has a policy for aerosol-generating procedures which says not to do certain things, but they don't follow it. We have suspected COVID patients on non-invasive ventilation who are on vented circuits, but they should be non-vented.

Nurse, medical specialty, female, age 31–40

Importance of being heard and in dialogue

Of great importance to healthcare workers was that the government and their employers recognised their expertise and listened to them. Healthcare workers wanted their experiences to be heard, validated, and acted on in meaningful ways.

I feel disregarded when the Chief Health Officer decides how I can effectively do my work without even discussing it with me.

Senior doctor, paediatrics, female, age 31–40

So much talk from the politicians. No true plan discussed with healthcare professionals. I would prefer we know the rationale behind certain decisions. No consultative approach. Poor communication.

General practitioner, female, age 51–64

Having leaders that listen to their staff, and implement feedback is really important. There is a lot of frustration when decisions are made that don't consider the needs of the healthcare workers. I think it's fine if all of our needs can't be met but it's important that they're considered, and if they can't be met that this is explained.

Physiotherapist, medical specialty, female, age 20–30

Often managers and administrators don't understand the nuances of clinical wards and why changes won't work. Listen to your staff, don't just tell them what to do. I appreciate that the Department of Health would pressure health managers, but they should be more transparent about decisions made.

Dietician, medical specialty, female, age 31–40

Good leaders support and look after their team. Unfortunately, many business leaders only get there by being ruthless and lacking in empathy. This probably has the greatest bearing on mental health and resilience of the team as staff need to feel respected, valued, and heard.

Senior doctor, radiology, male, age 41–50

Show healthcare workers they are listened to and validated. Not just heard and then vaguely remembered, no action.

Dentist, private practice, female, age 31–40

It is important to feel heard, appreciated, and looked after.

Speech pathologist, community care, female, age 20–30

I do think that managers need to listen to nurses who are working on the front and not just have forums where we can discuss our concerns. This does not work, and we are made to feel we are whining and not listened to. It makes us feel we are just a number, and it doesn't matter how many emails say we are doing a great job it doesn't mean a thing to me. I would like managers to be there for us and work with our concerns and not make us feel we are not coping.

Nurse, female, age 65–70

We have learnt not to suggest new ideas to our senior staff. They just do not listen. At the next staff meeting you just keep looking to the ground and agree.

Paramedic, male, age 51–64

Our voices will never reach anywhere anyway. We are too tired to even rise our voices.

Nurse, palliative care, female, age 41–50

Healthcare workers desired opportunities to have their concerns and ideas heard and respected.

> I would like the opportunity to be consulted about how I would prefer to work during the pandemic.
>
> *Social worker, palliative care, female, age 51–64*

> Provide personable communications with all staff. It would be amazing if the nurse unit manager could provide a contact for staff to debrief and reflect ideas on how we can improve our time during lengthy shifts when dealing with COVID.
>
> *Nurse, intensive care, female, age 41–50*

> There should be a channel to voice concerns and highlight issues to senior management.
>
> *Junior doctor, intensive care, male, age 31–40*

> Perhaps if government and hospital executives empowered frontline workers instead of impeding them, we could have handled this pandemic better?
>
> *Senior doctor, emergency department, female, age 31–40*

Videoconferencing and telehealth

Due to restrictions on face-to-face contact, telehealth was rapidly adopted as a primary way of providing healthcare. A suite of new regulatory and funding arrangements, including expanded government funding, facilitated the use of telephone or videoconferencing to deliver health services. Healthcare workers recognised the benefits of telehealth.

> COVID-19 has changed how we do our work. Some of it has been for the better. For example, telehealth has brought us up to the 21st century. I would really like it to continue beyond COVID-19 as a government-funded support, for metropolitan as well as for regional areas.
>
> *Psychologist, private practice, female, age 51–64*

> I've been lucky as the practice is mine and I could change to telehealth to protect myself and my patients.
>
> *Speech pathologist, community care, female, age 51–64*

However, the sudden change to using telehealth also generated challenges.

> The sudden shift to telehealth was great, but also challenging. Trying to see new patients on telehealth is really hard, almost a waste of their time. There

> is a hybrid clinic now of telehealth, face-to-face, and some by phone. I like to be fair and see people in order, but I cannot keep track of this in a public clinic. Some peers seem to stay in their consulting rooms, doing private work and not seeing patients, especially not seeing face-to-face patients. There are inequities.
>
> *Senior doctor, surgical, female, age 51–64*

> I feel the government should have helped more to provide GPs with the technology hardware to do video consults. It is a shame that it is mostly phone consults due to a lack of technology support.
>
> *General practitioner, female, age 65–70*

Healthcare workers told us how exhausting it was to spend full days carrying out online consultations.

> The shift to telehealth has had a big impact. I find it much more mentally draining and tiring to do a full day of patients via telehealth than in person.
>
> *Senior doctor, medical specialty, female, age 41–50*

> Lots of demand for psychology—via telehealth—causing some fatigue at times.
>
> *Psychologist, general medicine, female, age 31–40*

> Telehealth has been great, but it has expanded my hours too much. I'm using it mostly for follow-ups and simple presentations from known patients. But it's exhausting for me and time-consuming for staff.
>
> *General practitioner, female, age 51–64*

> I believe that it has been more tiring to consult via video than in person.
>
> *Psychologist, community care, female, age 41–50*

Some healthcare workers expressed concern that telehealth was inferior to face-to-face healthcare because of difficulties with ensuring patient privacy, detecting the nuances of verbal and non-verbal communication, and the impossibility of conducting physical assessments.

> There is a lot of emphasis on people working directly with COVID patients which is obviously important. However, there is little acknowledgement of healthcare workers who are trying to manage working from home using telehealth etc. This can be very challenging in the home environment, and patients are sometimes not receiving adequate care via telehealth which places a burden on the healthcare professional.
>
> *Dietitian, medical specialty, female, age 20–30*

> Telehealth training and clinical governance was absent, and we had to look to our rural colleagues for advice or overseas reports. We were very worried about telehealth being worse medicine than face-to-face in culturally and linguistically diverse, and Aboriginal and Torres Strait Islander communities due to communication, language, cultural challenges.
>
> *General practitioner, male, age 51–64*

> Telehealth services are not as effective or satisfying as face-to-face appointments.
>
> *Nurse, intensive care, female, age 41–50*

> I am aware of two confirmed cases of bowel cancer being diagnosed early, as the gastroenterologist continued to see her patients face-to-face and was able to examine patients. [With telehealth] the diagnosis would have been missed or delayed with a potentially poorer outcome for these two young people.
>
> *Senior doctor, paediatrics, female, age 41–50*

Social media

For some healthcare workers, social media was a lifeline—providing access to evolving information, the real-time experiences of international colleagues, and crucial social and collegial support. Several healthcare workers told us that the information they gleaned through Twitter and specialty-specific Facebook groups was more current and helpful than anything received through official channels. Along with Twitter, they particularly valued closed social media and messenger groups made up of healthcare workers with a shared area of interest.

> I've learnt more from the GPs Down Under Facebook group than from anywhere else, certainly nothing from any government organisations.
>
> *General practitioner, female, age 41–50*

> I've found Twitter and the COVID Doctors Facebook group useful.
>
> *Senior doctor, surgical, female, age 41–50*

> I have found more support on social media, especially Twitter, than I have from my workplace administration and area health service.
>
> *Senior doctor, emergency department, female, age 41–50*

> I don't know how I would have survived this pandemic without Twitter. So much collaboration and generosity in sharing and supporting each other on Twitter.
>
> *Speech pathologist, medical specialty, female, age 41–50*

> Our paediatric WhatsApp forum has been a godsend.
>
> *Senior doctor, medical specialty, female, age 51–64*

Not infrequently, the information shared on social media would be weeks or even months ahead of official government recommendations.

> A lot of guidance on COVID has come months after we have all had to sort out our own processes. I joined a Facebook page, GPs Down Under, and that has provided me with an enormous amount of timely information and support—100 times that of any other group supposed to be advising or assisting.
>
> *General practitioner, female, age 51–64*

> Getting an email, with the press release by our local public hospital, five days after we've already seen it on social media is ridiculous and devaluing.
>
> *Nurse, community care, female, age 51–64*

> The PPE discussions on social media platforms like Twitter from professionals (epidemiologists and infection control experts) who I respect, are anxiety provoking. I don't understand why if there is any level of uncertainty around aerosol generation from activities such as speech, why not openly discuss this, and take a more conservative approach, such as the use of N95 masks when working in closed room with a confirmed COVID-positive patient?
>
> *Allied health practitioner, intensive care, female, age 31–40*

However, social media had a downside too, as a vehicle for dangerously wrong information that eroded trust in health advice and public institutions. During the pandemic, the best parts of human nature were visibly present online, but so too were acts of ignorance, blame, and fear of the "other".

> Social media is very damaging. There are too many maniacs on Twitter with opinions that were unhelpful.
>
> *Senior doctor, anaesthetics, male, age 31–40*

> Conspiracy theories on social media have been a source of frustration, feeling defeated, and sometimes anxiety.
>
> *Junior doctor, general medicine, male, age 20–30*

> It is really hard when nufties share their opinion online to so many people and you cannot respond due to your job. It feels [like] the idiots can spread their silly opinions whilst those with knowledge are almost gagged due to trying to stay professional.
>
> *Nurse, intensive care, female, age 20–30*

> There are so many of the general public that are incredibly stupid but are very, very vocal about it on social media. It is so hard to keep going when friends, co-workers, and other people you know put out their desperate pleas, telling exactly how it is [caring for people with COVID], and people ridicule us and say we're liars or paid actors. It's hard to avoid, even when actively trying to disengage. It's so demoralising.
>
> *Nurse, medical specialty, female, age 31–40*

Traditional media

Media coverage of the pandemic was widely perceived by healthcare workers to be sensationalised.

> The media coverage has been unhelpful: inflammatory and sensationalist.
>
> *Nurse, surgical, female, age 41–50*

> I think it would be useful if the media stated facts instead of ramping things up.
>
> *Nurse, perioperative care, female, age 51–64*

> I'm sick of the media reporting false information, sick of hearing every five minutes about death tolls, sick of hearing "the worst day".
>
> *Nurse, emergency department, female, age 31–40*

> The excessive rubbish on television, causing controversy with others.
>
> *Nurse, hospital aged care, female, age 51–64*

> Our clinic felt that 90 percent of patients have taken the pandemic in their stride, obviously not enjoying it, but often taking the quieter home time as a positive. The media has not focused enough on how resilient people are and hence the public think 90 percent are suffering severely rather than 10 percent.
>
> *General practitioner, female, age 51–64*

Some healthcare workers worried about the impact of overblown media reports on the communities they served.

> If we had some way of moderating the sensationalised "news", the collateral damage on people's mental health would be mitigated.
>
> *Allied health practitioner, palliative care, female, age 51–64*

> I just wish the media didn't bombard the population with propaganda that makes our work harder.
>
> *General practitioner, female, age 51–64*

> The media warp the truth, and the community believe a lot of what they hear, and then are too worried and scared to attend health care services.
>
> *Nurse, emergency department, female, age 20–30*

Others raised concerns about the consequences of negative media portrayals of the healthcare sector and workforce.

> My current fear is that the media reports highlight current numbers which are related to healthcare workers. The impact of these reports is that the general public may feel that the health industry is slowing the economy and closing down jobs for them. Therefore, these reports in the media paint the health industry badly and as the bad guys, when the nature of this virus would be much worse if government lockdowns were not in place. Health care workers are very well educated on PPE and its use and contraction of the virus is often accidental. Negative reporting may cause a backlash. If so, how will the government react to this, and how will they support health care workers already being burnt out from their efforts?
>
> *Nurse, medical specialty, male, age 41–50*

> The media have a lot to answer for with regards to reporting personal information and identifying features regarding outbreaks and sources. Families and individuals made to feel shame and guilt, when most have simply done the best that they can in the situation they were in.
>
> *Nurse, community care, female, age 31–40*

Managing media exposure

Too much exposure—to either traditional or social media—was recognised as potentially harmful. Some healthcare workers told us that they turned off the television, and logged out of social media, as a way of managing the fear and stress provoked by endless coverage of coronavirus news. Others tried to curate a selection of reliable and trustworthy sources of information.

> Keeping perspective is an important strategy during this time. Not reading a lot of social media and being critical in approach to the information provided in the media so as not to take on everything at face value.
>
> *Nurse, intensive care, female, age 51–64*

> Facebook groups for doctors, like the doctors' COVID forum and the Medical Mums group, have been a source of helpful information but also can be anxiety provoking too.
>
> *Junior doctor, hospital aged care, female, age 20–30*

My wish list would be to reduce the media angst that is everywhere. I try and tune out, but my patients and friends and family pick up on it and the angst and anger it propagates.

General practitioner, female, age 51–64

History has shown us that disease will strike and cause chaos but [feeling] paralysed by media-driven fear is serving us negatively. In this day and age of instant access to information we see and hear too much, too soon, to our detriment.

Paramedic, male, age 41–50

11

FEELING VALUED AND APPRECIATED

> It takes many wheels and moving parts to keep hospitals and healthcare facilities moving. It's not just about the doctors and nurses—everyone from the cleaner to the CEO perform vital roles, and should be acknowledged as such, and not be an afterthought.
>
> *Nurse, hospital-based, female, age 51–64*

Few healthcare workers wanted to be lauded as heroes during the COVID-19 pandemic, but they did want to be valued and treated with respect. Healthcare workers wanted their workplaces to appreciate them and keep them safe. In this chapter we hear that gestures from workplaces were often viewed as "falling short", tokenistic, or invalidating by healthcare workers, unless they were accompanied by safe and fair working conditions. We also present views from different occupational groups—ranging from cleaners to laboratory technicians—who made crucial contributions to patient care, yet received little recognition for their work during the pandemic.

Authentic actions versus tokenistic gestures

Healthcare workers repeatedly expressed their frustration and disappointment over being offered personal wellbeing strategies, at a time when basic occupational health and safety protections in their workplaces were lacking. They saw this as shifting the responsibility for workplace health away from governments and health institutions onto individual members of the health workforce.

> I am angered by being constantly offered wellbeing programs by my employer and government authorities instead of full PPE with fit-testing and training. The elephant in the room is that I am worried about life-and-death survival

DOI: 10.4324/9781003228394-11

of me and my family from COVID-19 infection, and they want me to meditate and do crafts!

Administrative worker, medical specialty, female, age 51–64

I really think the most important thing is how Australia manages the COVID-19 pandemic and what our employer's attitude to occupational health and safety is. Everything else—all the individual level interventions like yoga apps—are chicken feed in comparison. There is a big risk that focusing on the individual-level strategies lets governments and employers "off the hook" and frames any distress as the worker's fault.

Junior doctor, psychiatry, male, age 31–40

We are the last line of defence, not the first. Calling us heroes is unreasonable. What is needed is a scientifically-safe environment for the patients and the workers. I feel that emergency medicine has not been taken seriously by the government.

Senior doctor, emergency department, male, age 51–64

Better workplaces need to be the priority, not simply Band-Aid yoga or mental health supports.

Junior doctor, paediatrics, female, age 20–30

It would be better if hospitals and executive management spent as much time focussing on practical solutions to the massive problems in infrastructure, staffing, and logistics in public hospitals, as on efforts to make us "feel better" about putting up with these outdated, inefficient, and incompetent systems. Don't just placate the staff or tell us about Lifeline or Beyond Blue. Fix the underlying problems that are causing the stress and distress.

Senior doctor, anaesthetics, female, age 41–50

For too long, healthcare workers have played up to the community expectation of "healthcare heroes and angels", which seems to relinquish the responsibility that our employers have to provide a safe workplace. I recall an early discussion, amongst senior staff, before the pandemic really kicked off in late February 2020. All had accepted that "at least a couple of us would get it". That sort of says it all. A complacency about workplace health and safety. Not one single healthcare worker should have got it at work.

Speech pathologist, oncology, female, age 41–50

Private hospitals are putting profits ahead of the pandemic. They seem to be trying to continue with a "business as usual" approach. They are showing little tangible regard for employee welfare. For example, giving out free coffee while denying masks, cutting hours, and still charging staff for parking.

Nurse, perioperative care, female, age 41–50

> You feel like you're trusted with responsibility, but the expectation is not met with appreciation or gratitude.
>
> *Physiotherapist, intensive care, female, age 20–30*

Some pointed out that small gestures offered to them by their employers diminished their role and their identity; particularly in the absence of monetary recognition, such as paid overtime or hazard pay.

> It feels like our hospital has been forgotten about, despite us working with the largest number of confirmed COVID-positive patients. We are working under very difficult circumstances, with 75 percent of staff per shift being bank or agency. We got a gift from the hospital: two squares of chocolate in an envelope. That's what we're worth apparently. We are all completely disillusioned with management now, we have no faith that they care about us.
>
> *Nurse, sub-acute aged care, female, age 31–40*

> I'm not feeling supported from the Federal Government. No hazard pay, just an empty "thank you" as frontline workers.
>
> *Nurse, intensive care, female, age 20–30*

> Healthcare workers risk their lives daily and that is stress that cannot be underestimated or overlooked. They deserve more than placatory words of praise. Financial security and bonuses help in times of emotional stress.
>
> *Senior doctor, emergency department, female, age 31–40*

> I want to be valued by organisations as a person whose opinion, life, and safety matters.
>
> *Senior doctor, anaesthetics, female, age 41–50*

> Can you imagine the bonuses executives would demand for dealing with something like this! We might get a chocolate frog if we are lucky. That is really what the community think of healthcare workers at the end of the day. We are a taxpayer burden until it's them [who needs care].
>
> *Nurse, intensive care, female, age 51–64*

However, depending on the context, small gestures were sometimes appreciated.

> Environmental services staff received a KitKat chocolate bar each. It was nice to be appreciated for the work we do in the hospitals everywhere. I don't think we are appreciated enough. It's a tough job cleaning the rooms of patients who have lost their fight with COVID, and passed on, or are positive and moved to the red [COVID-19] wards or ICU.
>
> *Hospital cleaner, female, age 51–64*

> Nice gestures, like a free coffee or chocolate from the community, was more positive exponentially than a recommendation to stay off alcohol and open another wellbeing app.
>
> *Junior doctor, medical specialty, male, age 31–40*

There was also frustration expressed when recognition was misdirected away from frontline healthcare workers.

> We need more acknowledgment from managers, medical teams, the public, and the government. We are on the frontline. We risk our young healthy bodies to help people get better from an illness that can't be cured. It frustrates me when managers get a lot of praise and they have never exposed themselves to a COVID patient by directly looking after them. It frustrates me that specific people always look after the COVID patients. We don't get enough recognition. We should get more recognition for sacrificing our own health, and our family's health.
>
> *Nurse, intensive care, female, age 31–40*

Messages that superficially appeared to be supportive and caring, were sometimes perceived as silencing healthcare workers from speaking out about safety concerns.

> Applause and open letters from the Premier mean next to nothing to me and other people I know … All this achieves is shaming public workers into not speaking out about their frustrations because we've been pushed into this frontline "hero" role that none of us asked to be in or agreed to.
>
> *Junior doctor, intensive care, male, age 20–30*

> There appeared to be a lot of talk about protecting frontline staff but small follow through. Many of us were "silenced" for having opinions other than the status quo. This isolated me even more.
>
> *Nurse, respiratory medicine, female, age 51–64*

> Managers throw emailed platitudes around, but many on-floor staff express that they do not feel supported. Face-to-face (1.5 metre distance) is truly required, it's what we give our patients and each other, but hardly ever receive ourselves from middle management. Empty platitudes grate on our senses.
>
> *Nurse, medical specialty, female, age 51–64*

> The mixed messaging from my direct manager is very disappointing. Writing all the right things in emails but—in reality—the care factor about staff is minimal.
>
> *Respiratory scientist, female, age 41–50*

> I just wish they stopped referring to us as "heroes". There is nothing heroic about what we do. I also find it irritatingly annoying and anger-provoking when tertiary hospitals are using this pandemic to beg for donations.
>
> *Senior doctor, emergency department, male, age 51–64*

> We feel we are being patted on the head like we are children. I've had a gutful.
>
> *Nurse, perioperative care, female, age 51–64*

> No one is actually there to support. Everyone seems to offer support, until you ask for it. Then they offer nothing.
>
> *Junior doctor, emergency department, male, age 31–40*

Feeling forgotten

Many healthcare workers felt unseen, unheard, and overlooked, particularly as the pandemic went on and public support waned. This evoked feelings of disappointment and disillusionment for many.

Some said that the entire frontline workforce was under-appreciated.

> We are all equally undervalued and disposable in our health system.
>
> *Senior doctor, medical specialty, female, age 31–40*

Others felt that certain occupations and work areas were valued less than high profile areas such as the intensive care units and infectious diseases wards of major hospitals; even though they were also experiencing similar work pressures and exposing themselves to risk every day.

> It does seem like some areas are more important, like some people's jobs are not as valued. That is a strong message that is hard to ignore when you are in that environment. Not everyone is treated equally!
>
> *Nurse, medical specialty, female, age 51–64*

> This saturated attention on the "glamorous" areas of the hospital pulled at my sense of worth as a nurse, having personally encountered the plight of my fellow colleagues battling COVID in areas of nursing that may not appeal to the public eye.
>
> *Nurse, surgical, female, age 31–40*

> I felt the organisation I work with showed favouritism towards some healthcare workers over others which further made me feel frustrated and at times useless. Especially when all you want to do is help!
>
> *Nurse, casual pool, female, age 51–64*

> Some staff groups have been singled out to receive support in the form of care packages. This causes division amongst work groups and creates an "us and them" mentality.
>
> *Administrative worker, general medicine, female, age 51–64*

> Double standards. The administration protected some people from doing too much, or being potentially exposed to COVID-19, whilst others were put at extra risk.
>
> *Senior doctor, palliative care, female, age 41–50*

> I wish there had been more support for the sub-acute wards. Intensive care units and infectious disease wards were getting support and fanfare every day. Our sub-acute ward—that became a 25-bed fully COVID-positive ward—has barely been mentioned.
>
> *Nurse, sub-acute aged care, female, age 31–40*

> Few thoughts are given to those delivering services to mental health patients. All accolades are given to doctors and nurses, not counsellors and psychologists who are working directly with those suffering in the communities.
>
> *Social worker, community care, female, age 51–64*

> Everyone is super aware of the risk doctors and nurses face. However, the people that facilitate them are ignored. From front-desk workers or security or facilities/building management, through to orderlies and medical imaging staff. All these people face risk and they don't get free coffee or applauded or even thanked.
>
> *Dental therapist, emergency dental, female, age 20–30*

Community and primary care

There was perceived to be little recognition for the risks experienced by healthcare workers who were the first point of contact for patients in the community, including pharmacists, dentists, general practitioners, disability support workers, and other healthcare providers in community and primary care.

> My job in dental is patient-facing and we worked through COVID to keep dental pain patients out of waiting rooms and reduce people overloading general care. We aren't lifesavers but our job was important.
>
> *Dental therapist, emergency dental, female, age 20–30*

> Pharmacists are an important and vital part of the health care system. In community we deal with referring patients every day to the screening clinic

and in most circumstances are the first port of call to provide vital public health information. Where is our PPE? We vaccinated the population from the flu and now are looking at a plan for how to educate patients on COVID symptoms during allergy season. Support is needed!

Pharmacist, community care, female, age 31–40

Pharmacists are underutilised and underappreciated. We are on the frontline giving advice about general health and specific pandemic protection measures, as well as navigating our regular roles under new restrictions.

Pharmacist, community care, female, age 20–30

Pharmacists are often left out of the frontline worker category. However, we are the ones who people come to see as soon as they have a scratchy sore throat or headache or cough before they believe their symptoms are "serious enough" for a COVID test. It has been frustrating that this is rarely acknowledged.

Pharmacist, community care, female, age 31–40

COVID-19 has had a massive impact on pharmacists and pharmacy staff. We have been under the pump throughout this crisis with little-to-no support from the health department. It feels like we are under-appreciated in comparison to other health professions and get forgotten about as front-line health professionals. We deal with sick patients closely everyday with no PPE most of the time.

Pharmacist, community care, female, age 20–30

Pharmacists have been significantly impacted but are often not considered to be frontline workers even though they have to remain on duty and deal with the public every day. People come to the pharmacy with symptoms that may be COVID-19 seeking treatment when they are supposed to be in isolation or before they are tested.

Pharmacist, community care, female, age 51–64

Primary care is regarded as an essential fundamental service when it comes to availability of appointments and timely access, moral obligations and duty of care. But when it comes to supply of PPE or funding for adaptation, it's left to fend for itself with scraps.

General practitioner, male, age 31–40

I strongly feel that GPs could have been more involved in testing and tracing—we were actually doing this work—it was just off the record and unrecognised. What a shame that we—the primary care providers—have once again been overlooked. Yet we remain the most cost-effective aspect of the health system! Oh, and if we were funded properly to provide medical care in aged care facilities, maybe we wouldn't have the disastrous outbreaks we have seen!

General practitioner, female, age 41–50

Support from politicians and the media is important. Not the "hero" line, but the absence of vilification. Personally, my own anxiety skyrocketed when Dr Chris Higgins [a GP who contracted COVID-19] was treated the way he was by both politicians and media. It made me feel that I was exposing myself to significant risk (risks of Telehealth, risks of contracting COVID) for a system that would not hesitate to use me as a scapegoat. GPs have been left out of the system response at a time when they could have enhanced the response. There was very little access to PPE. I am incredibly lucky to be in a practice who have sourced their own at significant expense but not all were so lucky.

General practitioner, female, age 31–40

Allied health were left in the cold for ages. I'm 30cm from a patient's face and no one cared about us. Departments of Health only cared about registered allied health professions like physiotherapists (who actually aren't even as close as us touching faces and eyes and patients breathing on us).

Orthoptist, private practice, female, age 51–64

Community workers were, and still are, visiting clients in their homes so are at high risk.

Occupational therapist, community care, female, age 51–64

Support staff

Cleaners, kitchen staff, and facilities staff faced greater workloads due to the demands for more frequent and intensive cleaning. Those working in wards with COVID-positive patients were also at increased risk of infection.

We're all in this together in the hospital, not just doctors and nurses. I am a cleaner and we clean the rooms and the waste every day. Every worker in the hospital should be looked after.

Hospital cleaner, male, age 51–64

Please acknowledge the cleaning, catering, and maintenance staff as frontline workers. We can be exposed to COVID as well, not just the doctors and nurses.

Support staff, hospital-based, female, age 20–30

COVID-19 has impacted everyone's life who works in the same department and hospital that I do. You have to isolate yourself from your loved ones to keep them safe. It is stressful when you, and all the staff around you, are doing

> everything they can to keep themselves the community and their families safe and you see people outside of work just being complete a**holes.
>
> *Hospital cleaner, female, age 51–64*

> I have watched clinical decisions get made with cleaners and patient support assistants completely undervalued and under-resourced due to a lack of understanding of clinical care across a variety of settings.
>
> *Nurse, infectious diseases, female, age 41–50*

> We need more inclusion and support for the people who keep us safe: the cleaners, the garbage disposal workforce, the kitchen staff.
>
> *Senior doctor, medical specialty, female, age 51–64*

Patient transport staff also faced new workplace challenges.

> We are looked down on because we are "patient transport". Patient transport wages are less than a dog groomer. We have been working our asses off, while watching the government pay people almost the same pay for sitting on their couch safe at home all day. We have put our lives at risk and our families, not knowing what we are walking into on a job. When we transport a confirmed COVID patient we are told to wear an apron, with our pants exposed, and then get sent straight to another job in the same clothes. We are not treated equally. We need to be looked after!
>
> *Patient transport, female, age 20–30*

Clerical and administrative staff

Clerical and administrative staff were the first point of contact for patients and families and played a central role in keeping wards and clinics running. They struggled with increased demands, rising distress among patients and families, and technology that was never designed to support working from home.

> Everyone thanks the doctors and the nurses, but the administrative workers are never acknowledged. Our work is important also.
>
> *Administrative worker, emergency department, female, age 51–64*

> I would love to see investment in the support and training of administration and other non-clinical staff. I'd be interested to see how many healthcare worker infections—and consequent community transmissions—could have been prevented if better support was offered. I really can't overstate how disappointing this experience has been, I feel like myself and colleagues in similar roles have been completely forgotten.
>
> *Administrative worker, radiology, female, age 31–40*

As the ward clerk, I'm the first point of contact for many people. I haven't even been asked how things are going by my supervisor. Being continually abused over visitor restrictions was so stressful and is still continuing.

Ward clerk, general medicine, female, age 51–64

I am working much longer hours, due to the technology I am using not being suited to the task, making my work difficult. I am exhausted trying to maintain the output while dealing with IT issues. I am struggling to stay in the job. I feel the care for team members does not include me.

Administrative worker, female, age 51–64

I manage five different specialist clinics. There are around 90 doctors' lists per week to action. All these appointments needed to be changed. My workload increased but my paid hours didn't. I had to either come to work early, or finish late, to keep up. The hospital's priority was not, I felt, supporting the administrative staff. We had to fight for Perspex glass in clinics, for masks, goggles, and other equipment. I felt we were always one step behind.

Administrative worker, female, age 51–64

A hospital is not made up of doctors and nurses. There's a whole team of other unsung heroes who go to work day-in day-out leaving their family to keep this place going!

Administrative worker, female, age 51–64

Laboratory and radiology staff

Laboratory workers played a central role in the pandemic response, processing many tens of thousands of COVID-19 tests a day whenever outbreaks occurred.

We faced extra pressure from management and the Department of Health to get tests done and timely reporting. The mood in the laboratory was down. It would have helped if management understood the pressure we were under and arranged extra cover to help with the workload.

Senior doctor, pathology, female, age 41–50

Pathology staff should not be so overlooked by government, hospitals and other health care workers. Without us, you don't get your test results.

Laboratory technician, pathology, male, age 31–40

I was one of the few people in the laboratory able to perform COVID testing. Before COVID we were conducting around 96 PCR tests a day across the testing board. At the height of testing, we were performing 800

> plus per day. Doctors and nurses from across the hospital would routinely call and abuse staff for not having their own result or their patient's results yet.
>
> *Laboratory technician, pathology, male, age 31–40*

Radiographers also didn't feel valued as frontline staff.

> As a radiographer in Australia, we are not really deemed frontline by most people, including the public and media. It's hard to be in full PPE in the emergency department or intensive care and be overlooked by many.
>
> *Radiographer, emergency department, female, age 51–64*

Junior doctors

During the pandemic, workplace demands increased for many junior doctors. At the same time, they were still required to compete for places on specialist training programs and study for specialty exams, which were changed or cancelled at short notice during the pandemic.

> Our years and years of study and career progression goals have been thrown into uncertainty.
>
> *Junior doctor, general medicine, female, age 20–30*

> It would help if the [medical specialty] Colleges would communicate more openly and be more generous with trainees in this unprecedented situation.
>
> *Junior doctor, medical specialty, female, age 31–40*

> The impact on specialty exam processes and preparation has been the most important issue for me as I am sitting my primary exam and have been unable to prepare in the normal way. Preparation courses have been cancelled and communication from my college about the exam timing and process has been poor.
>
> *Junior doctor, intensive care, female, age 20–30*

> I'm currently studying for physicians' exams with the Royal Australasian College of Physicians. As Victorians, we felt completely blindsided by the College's lack of communication and lack of emotional support with the cancellation and re-scheduling of a virtual exam. It feels as though senior doctors are sometimes completely out of touch with the work and emotional stress on their junior colleagues. This has led to a lot of anger towards the hierarchal medical system.
>
> *Junior doctor, general medicine, male, age 20–30*

> The main contributor to my stress has been impending Basic Physician Trainee [specialist medical] clinical exam: how it will be run? how can I see

patients? what it will mean for jobs next year? Timely and effective communication from the College would help.

Junior doctor, hospital aged care, female, age 31–40

We have been affected by poor management of trainee trajectory and exams through COVID. More College support—not just statements but real support—would be helpful.

Junior doctor, community mental health, female, age 31–40

Our [specialist medical] exam was delayed with little communication, no change to the exam fee, and little information about the new format.

Junior doctor, medical specialty, female, age 31–40

Trainee supervisors need more time to teach and supervise and support junior staff.

Senior doctor, emergency department, female, age 41–50

Students

Similarly, healthcare students expressed concern about lost learning opportunities, disruption to placements, and poor communication from education providers.

Reduced placement times reduced preparedness for next year, with dramatically disturbed learning opportunities this year.

Student, surgical, female, age 20–30

I'm about to begin working as an intern at a busy hospital. I'm concerned about being an incompetent doctor. I'm really frightened about not being capable, and I generally consider myself able to appraise my skill set fairly.

Final year medical student, surgical, female, age 20–30

Too often we didn't receive information from the hospital we were placed at because students are excluded from the usual staff information sources. During the height of the second lockdown, while things were changing daily, it would have been useful to receive that information before we went onto the wards.

Student, palliative care, female, age 20–30

The university I attend as a medical student contributed majorly to my anxiety and depression. They were unsupportive, and inflexible. They assume all their medical students have the luxury of living at home with mum and dad and can come into placements at the drop of a hat. So many of us were struggling. Yet, when we reached out for help, they would threaten us with not graduating on time. They extended placements. They were unforgiving. They added more and more assessments. It was awful.

Medical student, intensive care, female, age 20–30

As students we were pulled out of placements and hence were not able to contribute and learn our work as previously. In the event of a future pandemic, a more inclusive approach to students who are eager to be there and help out would be appreciated.

Student, male, age 31–40

As students we are meant to be informed by the clinical school about what is happening within the hospital. However, we have often only heard second- or third-hand, if at all, regarding changes or potential exposures etc. It certainly feels like students have been forgotten which is concerning. As final year medical students, we have been asked to assist teams and keep them running with staff getting furloughed, but we don't receive the additional communication needed to keep us safe. Please support final year medical students who are helping on the wards. We are willing to help, but include us in conversations and communication as being in the dark is a source of stress for many.

Student, emergency department, male, age 20–30

Train students to be active members of clinical teams, not pot plants, so that next time we will be ready to be useful members of clinical teams!

Student, general medicine, male, age 20–30

The need for genuine appreciation and support

Many healthcare workers wrote about the need for meaningful support from their employers and managers.

Most of us just want to feel appreciated. And less of a commodity.

Medical scientist, emergency department, female, age 31–40

I feel like the public appreciated our efforts more than our employers did.

Nurse, hospital aged care, female, age 51–64

Was fed up being asked very frequently by kind well-meaning cold-zone [non-COVID ward/area] people in management how was I feeling. They simply had no way of understanding with empathy how bad it really was on the floor. Got fed up that the response seemed to always be the offering of the wellbeing phone number. What would've helped more was enough staff on the floor to enable breaks to be taken for as long as needed to regain hydration and equilibrium.

Nurse, hospital aged care, female, age 51–64

> Surely in this time we should be supplying scrubs and showering facilities for staff. We should be getting free parking and those working in high-risk COVID areas like ED, ICU, fever clinics, respiratory units and primary healthcare should be having their meals supplied and at least 15 minutes extra pre-break time.
>
> *Nurse, emergency department and primary care, female, age 51–64*

> During the pandemic, a close family member—not of the same household—contracted the virus which placed an additional set of emotional stressors on me. Whilst I received initial support and check-ins the first week, upon coming back to work, I received no support or check-in from my management, which made me feel as though they had only initially checked in to "tick some boxes" and determine whether I would be in quarantine. That family member suffered from a severe form of the virus and was in ICU for two weeks and I was required to quarantine for two weeks as well. After an experience like this, as I'm sure many other health professionals have been through, it would be great if management checked-in on staff. Even afterwards, as those who have gone through a situation like this are still experiencing the after-effects.
>
> *Radiographer, emergency department, female, age 20–30*

> Managers forget the fundamental reason we come to work is to make a difference in the life of those most vulnerable and in need. However they lack the basic social skills to show appreciation and thanks to their hard-working staff. A little thanks goes a long way and can fundamentally change your attitude towards work if you feel valued and appreciated. Sadly this seems to be lost on managers or done in a tokenistic and disingenuous way.
>
> *Social worker, medical specialty, female, age 20–30*

The importance of emotional validation

Healthcare workers said they found it comforting to have their feelings validated by others, including feelings of shame or hopelessness.

> Having feelings validated by others. It's strangely comforting that others are feeling the same as me, even though the feelings are really deflating and uncomfortable.
>
> *Dietician, general medicine, female, age 20–30*

> I would have appreciated knowing that other people were also feeling "low" and "flat" and that these were valid responses to the situation.
>
> *Physiotherapist, research unit, female, age 51–64*

> Having people listen without judgement or giving advice is great.
>
> *Medical imaging, community care, female, age 31–40*

Positive support that there is no shame to feeling burnt out or being tired.

Nurse, emergency department, female, age 20–30

Just knowing that we're all going through the same crazy time, and there's lots of people feeling anxious like me. That can be validating.

Social worker, community care, female, age 41–50

As a junior doctor, acts of kindness and understanding from senior staff and faculty really help.

Junior doctor, medical specialty, female, age 20–30

I had not worked with patients who were dying before. That changed very rapidly with COVID. Being able to hear my sadness acknowledged by senior staff was immensely helpful.

Student nurse, general medicine, female, age 31–40

None of us asked for this, or expected it, or volunteered for it, but we have to work in it … Validating those feelings, and not trying to steamroll them with positivity, is helpful.

Music therapist, palliative care, female, age 20–30

12

SHOWING UP ALL THE CRACKS

> The pandemic has shown up all the cracks in a chronically dysfunctional health care system.
>
> *Senior doctor, anaesthetics, female, age 51–64*

The COVID-19 pandemic widened existing disparities within society and within in the healthcare system, with profound consequences for patients and practitioners. In this chapter, healthcare workers describe how the problems encountered during the pandemic are inextricably linked with long-standing deficits and inequities in the healthcare system. These include an inequitable distribution of resources across localities, professions, and care sectors; an underpaid, overworked, and casualised workforce; and out-of-date technologies and systems. As healthcare workers explain, the experience of the pandemic differed between those with authority and power, and those who were marginalised and disempowered. Healthcare workers argued that these problems were amplified, not created, by the pandemic and they wrote about the urgent need to fix these longstanding problems.

Amplifying the deficiencies that already existed

Many healthcare workers expressed concern that known shortcomings in the healthcare system were magnified during the pandemic. An over-reliance on an underfunded and overstretched workforce and system was one key concern.

> The issues that were in the workplace before, have just been magnified by the pandemic.
>
> *Nurse, community care, female, age 51–64*

DOI: 10.4324/9781003228394-12

> COVID hasn't caused any new problems, it has merely highlighted all the pre-existing inadequacies of the healthcare system and society in general.
>
> *Senior doctor, emergency department, female, age 31–40*

> The impact of COVID has amplified the shortcomings of a healthcare system that lacks resources. The hospital is often run overcapacity and these problems have not been addressed pre-COVID. Better working conditions and an increase in resources is needed.
>
> *Radiographer, emergency department, female, age 20–30*

> We need more nursing staff and improved patient ratios.
>
> *Nurse, emergency department, female, age 31–40*

> The pandemic has merely exposed the pre-existing issues we were struggling with. Colleagues who were highly supportive are even more so, the behaviour of those who were draining or difficult in teams deteriorated. Shortages of staff and resources worsened. Lack of leave and unpaid overtime worsened. The drain on limited services to provide education to junior staff and students has worsened due to the increased clinical load. The only resource we had, that we could increase, was personal sacrifice of our own wellbeing. And the systems don't seem to have acknowledged the pre-existing nature of these issues.
>
> *Senior doctor, palliative care, female, age 41–50*

Healthcare workers wrote that they were angered and frustrated that there was an expectation on them, individually and as a group, to hold up a fractured system through working harder, "making do", and self-sacrifice.

> Everyone is trying their best in what is a crazy challenging time and Australia is doing well. But our strong and resilient healthcare workers cannot continue to hold up a fractured health system without more support and meaningful change, so that we can work in safe workplaces and feel the state and federal health departments have our back. Telehealth has been a massive win but delays in PPE-resourcing and appropriateness, testing, reporting, and contact tracing six months into the pandemic have been unacceptable and soul destroying. Our response to stopping a third wave is only as strong as the support we give in keeping our healthcare workers safe and aiming for elimination. Healthcare workers are not robots that are expendable for the sake of the economy. Without a strong safe health system we have no economy.
>
> *Senior doctor, medical specialty, male, age 41–50*

> Funding to health care has been underwhelming for too long. At my hospital, the attitude of "we must make-do" is highly lauded. Whilst the ability to

"make-do" is useful, when it comes to our healthcare systems, we should not have to merely "make-do".

Nurse, perioperative care, female, age 31–40

Medicine as a profession is already mostly short-staffed, especially in smaller hospitals. On good days, we are already stretched, stretching ourselves to do more and more. When something stressful like a pandemic or disaster happens, we are expected to put in even more hours plus the extra stress. There is no buffer.

Junior doctor, hospital aged care, female, age 20–30

A casualised workforce

Far from affecting healthcare workers equally, the burden of COVID-19 was unevenly distributed according to deeply entrenched inequities. Several outbreaks in Australia were linked to casual staff who were working across multiple sites due to low pay and a lack of job security.

I am part-time and casual and not a regular member of a team. I find that there is little support, as so much of the support and information is provided through permanent workplace teams.

Nurse, general medicine, female, age 51–64

Casual hospital employees have taken a huge hit, no-one ever says "thank you".

Administrative worker, infectious diseases, female, age 51–64

Casuals feel cut off from the hospital information stream.

Pharmacist, emergency department, female, age 31–40

I work on the nurse bank and don't have a regular team or colleagues to debrief with. I worked a number of shifts (every weekend for approximately six weeks) on the COVID wards and never had any follow up or connection with staff.

Nurse, general medicine, female, age 20–30

Because I was casual, it wasn't clear what level of pay I would receive if I had to isolate.

Nurse, emergency department, female, age 20–30

After being casually employed for seven years, I was suddenly unable to get any work at my hospital. How is it possible that a huge public hospital can have no shifts for loyal bank staff, and totally desert us so easily?

Nurse, maternity, female, age 41–50

> I was sent into an aged care home as an agency nurse, with no handover, no guidance as to exactly what my role was to be. It was chaotic, and disorganised, and made me feel very unsafe.
>
> *Nurse, residential aged care, female, age 51–64*

> It would be helpful to have more support for casual staff.
>
> *Nurse, emergency department, female, age 20–30*

Shift workers also pointed to inequities in training and resources for night shift workers compared with the day shift.

> Please remember night shift, we do work here as well!
>
> *Support staff, hospital-based, female, age 20–30*

> Remember there are night staff that are affected. Changes in protocols and processes are focused around daytime activities. There's been very little information given that is focused on the effects on night shift workers, which a lot of health workers are.
>
> *Sleep scientist, respiratory medicine, female, age 31–40*

> As I work nights, I never see my boss and she has never once emailed or messaged to see how her night staff are.
>
> *Administrative worker, emergency department, female, age 41–50*

> My partner lost his job, so the children were not permitted to attend childcare, which meant sleeping after night shift was impossible.
>
> *Nurse, general medicine, female, age 41–50*

> Night shift staff weren't given proper, face-to-face PPE instruction from a person in a senior or experienced clinical role: we were "instructed" on PPE by outgoing clerical staff who were just in a rush to get home.
>
> *Administrative worker, emergency department, female, age 31–40*

Job insecurity was of particular concern, especially for lower-paid and more junior staff.

> Job security needs to be taken seriously. We need better support for support workers, pharmacists, dieticians, etc not just nurses.
>
> *Nurse, medical specialty, male, age 41–50*

> The lack of job security for junior doctors has always been a problem but has been exacerbated by the pandemic.
>
> *Junior doctor, surgical, male, age 31–40*

> Because of the delay in junior staff being able to progress onto the next stage, there is then limited job availability for next year. With the threat of not having a job next year, people are anxious and worried about their career viability.
>
> *Junior doctor, general medicine, female, age 41–50*

> Many of my friends and colleagues have found the annual job search and attempt to get on to training programs even more unbearable and non-transparent than usual this year.
>
> *Junior doctor, surgical, male, age 31–40*

Overlooking regional healthcare

While most COVID-19 infections occurred in cities, regional and rural areas of Australia struggled too. Services in these areas are often under-funded and short-staffed and were already buckling after the devastating bushfires that swept through the summer before the pandemic began.

> Regional Victoria has been a bit forgotten. There's been a lot of focus on metro areas but huge risk factors if COVID spreads to smaller towns and impacts on smaller communities.
>
> *Nurse, community care, female, age 41–50*

> It's been a long hard slog in rural areas with small staff numbers. Every time someone goes off for COVID testing, and it takes a few days to get results, someone else has to fill their shifts. We have no agency or casuals.
>
> *Nurse, community care, female, age 41–50*

> I work in a regional hospital which has 10 to 25 patients in isolation at a time awaiting COVID clearance. It's not just a positive test that affects care, so does awaiting a negative.
>
> *Junior doctor, female, age 20–30*

> My department is chronically underfunded—we have had three vacancies without those positions being covered for months—and rather than acknowledge these systemic challenges, managers make it out like there is something wrong with us: "not working fast enough … not coping well enough".
>
> *Social worker, medical specialty, female, age 20–30*

> Small health services don't have access to the supports of larger services. Our residents were suffering, and we needed more resources to keep them connected. We had dedicated leaders who walked the talk and stayed connected with staff. But we didn't have any extra workforce to implement all the new ideas and changes.
>
> *Nurse, hospital aged care, female, age 51–64*

> There was no free coffee, hampers, or pizza for nurses working with COVID patients in Regional Victoria. Just more unpaid overtime.
>
> *Nurse, community care, male, age 51–64*

> Rural urgent care centres have been expected to take on an increased work load with little or no increase in staff. The physical setting limitations have meant that we are expected to look after patients in two different areas as in hot [COVID] and cold [non-COVID] zones with just two nursing staff and one doctor, making infection control guidelines almost impossible to maintain. When concerns are expressed, there has been little or no effective response.
>
> *Nurse, emergency department, female, age 51–64*

> So far, COVID-19 has had much less impact in regional Australia than in the cities, so it has been more of a nuisance than a threat. But public health needs to take spread to regional areas seriously. We don't have the resources to cope if there is a significant outbreak.
>
> *General practitioner, female, age 41–50*

Aged care: neglected and forgotten

The under-funded and under-resourced aged care sector was written about at length. Healthcare workers were particularly concerned about the disproportionate burden of COVID-19 infections and deaths in aged care settings and the need for additional resources to be allocated to the sector.

> There is a lot of waiting in aged care—waiting to see if COVID will happen in your organisation. This really affects the quality of life of the residents, and staff need to spend more time with them to make up for no family visits and social isolation. Additional staff need to be allocated at times of a pandemic to meet this additional emotional/social need. Aged care funding should reflect this.
>
> *Administrative worker, residential aged care, female, age 51–64*

> Our residents are missing day centre, exercise groups and bus outings. Even pets have not been allowed to visit them; for some older people the pets keep them going.
>
> *Nurse, hospital aged care, female, age 31–40*

> Aged care needs an overhaul as many centres are money-makers alone.
>
> *Nurse, surgical, female, age 51–64*

> If it were children who were worst affected by this virus, we would not be having these callous discussions about opening up the economy and borders

early. Stop devaluing the lives of older people. The older people who are stranded in hospital post COVID-19 infection are often dying from iatrogenic harm from being in hospital. We need a strategy to manage these people in a more residential environment.

Physiotherapist, general medicine, male, age 31–40

Every healthcare worker I know … actually everyone I know was horrified by the events at a certain residential aged care facility. The delay in taking decisive action was appalling, as was Ministers blaming the staff member who allegedly was "patient zero". I fully appreciate that deaths occur in aged care facilities, but the management of the situation was disastrous. Seriously it took HOW LONG to take appropriate measures? I have also held considerable fears for the staff working in that organisation and I sincerely hope ALL supportive measures were put in place … and NO I don't mean … "here's the number you can call if you're feeling stressed".

Nurse, palliative care, female, age 51–64

The aged care sector needs closer scrutiny, as what has been happening there for many years puts not only the residents but also the whole community at risk. We are all going to get old at some point and we need to ensure this sector improves. More registered nurses are needed to supervise the patient care attendants who are ill-equipped to detect many health problems and obviously have not been adequately trained in PPE use.

Nurse, perioperative care, female, age 51–64

We need to value aged care workers as a specialty more to reflect the complexity of our work.

Nurse, residential aged care, female, age 51–64

We need a to start enacting changes to how geriatric patient care is delivered in long term care facilities alongside improving community supports to reduce unnecessary institutionalisation. The skills of the workforce, for aged care in residential care facilities, are in dire need of up-skilling and infection control design needs to be examined.

Junior doctor, hospital aged care, female, age 31–40

Most of Australia's deaths have been in people from aged care, so managing these outbreaks in a timelier manner would have prevented many deaths.

Nurse, medical specialty, female, age 51–64

I have worked at two aged care residences with COVID outbreaks for a total of about three months. We have sadly had 20 clients lose their lives and dealt with over 100 cases from staff and residents. I feel there has been so much negativity on how aged care coped throughout the pandemic and I don't feel this is the case for all outbreaks aged care services experienced. I heard nothing but positive and upbeat comments from outreach teams throughout. They were often there to see if there was anything they could do to assist and to check on our progress which we were grateful for but also at times providing conflicting information. We thanked them for this often with a smile when inside we were more confused. I have since seen some of those exact people speaking about all the negative things they experienced during the outbreak in aged care and not one of the positives. It would help a lot of us who work in aged care to not feel like COVID deaths and complications are directly our fault which sadly sometimes this is exactly how we feel.

Nurse, residential aged care, female, age 31–40

Every time that I hear a person over 100 years old has died from COVID, I weep.

Nurse, palliative care, female, age 51–64

For a while my role was ensuring "all the boxes were ticked" before transferring bodies to the morgue.

Nurse, hospital aged care, female, age 51–64

Compensation and hazard pay

Many healthcare workers, particularly nurses, wrote about being underpaid. They conveyed their disappointment that the critical value of their roles during the pandemic had not translated into any financial recognition or reward. A number called for "hazard pay" to compensate for the high risks associated with their work during the pandemic.

I think all frontline workers should be getting hazard pay, especially nursing staff. We are working in an extremely high-risk position, and we don't get any extra for doing it, we are placing our families at risk.

Nurse, general medicine, female, age 20–30

We nurses are not paid enough to deal with this.

Nurse, surgical, female, age 41–50

We should be getting danger money. We are putting our health at risk to deal with a deadly respiratory virus using plastic aprons and masks.

Nurse, medical specialty, male, age 20–30

Honestly, I know this might not ever happen but some sort of financial benefit would help. We always put our lives at risk; however this time is more dangerous and serious than ever.

Nurse, intensive care, female, age 20–30

I only worked in the COVID clinic for a few weeks, but my nursing colleagues with young children and elderly parents have been there for over half a year now. They should be rewarded with hazard pay for everything they do to keep the public safe.

Junior doctor, medical specialty, female, age 20–30

I do feel there should be some bonus pay or pandemic allowance for people working closely with COVID patients as it will make them less worried financially if something bad should happen to them.

Nurse, emergency department, female, age 41–50

It seems the economy has spent on many other things, except rewarding nurses who have had to go on and experience higher levels of stress and fatigue than anyone. It sometimes brings about feelings of resentment.

Nurse, palliative care, female, age 41–50

The public certainly think we get paid more than we do. We nurses are so underpaid it's a joke. Better pay would help.

Nurse, respiratory medicine, female, age 20–30

I felt completely upset when I found out the traffic control staff on construction sites earn more than most senior nurses.

Nurse, infectious diseases, female, age 51–64

We should not be out of pocket for our efforts. This has been a real bug bear for me. I have had to buy extra shoes to leave at work, and other essentials, and none of this has been covered. It is not good enough. With all the donning and doffing, and car parks turned into lunch rooms, my 9 hour days are now 10.5 hour days. And to not be offered any compensation for this is not fair. Money isn't everything but it can pay for face cream under masks and an extra pair of shoes that wouldn't be needed if I wasn't doing my bit.

Nurse, general medicine, female, age 51–64

I feel like nursing staff have been very underappreciated and that there is little understanding how hard we work. I see politicians earning large sums of money and it's quite obvious who works the hardest when times are tough. We are underpaid and undervalued and if we aren't careful, we won't have a workforce left.

Nurse, surgical, female, age 31–40

I feel nursing staff have been thrown into this and there has been more support given to doctors, yet they are in the infectious area less than half the time. I have heard a consultant say it "wasn't fair" that her interns had to stay

> in a HOT [COVID ward] zone and wear PPE all shift. Um, well as nurses that's what we have to do, so why should it be any different for doctors.
>
> *Nurse, general medicine, female, age 31–40*

> We are told by some we are heroes, yet I'm probably never going to be able to afford a house on my current nurse's wage. Kind words are nice but a pay rise would be nicer.
>
> *Nurse, infectious disease, female, age 20–30*

The heavy burden on junior staff

Some healthcare workers, especially junior doctors, described the heavy burden being placed on the junior workforce. Their concerns about excessive workloads, exhausting rosters, unpaid overtime, and training needs being subsumed to service requirements all reflected an exacerbation of pre-existing problems.

> There is minimal acknowledgement from hospitals that the burden is placed unequally towards junior medical staff.
>
> *Junior doctor, general medicine, male, age 20–30*

> Junior staff cover COVID wards every week whereas many senior staff now conduct only paper rounds [where patients are discussed without visiting the patient's bedside] to limit exposure to COVID patients.
>
> *Junior doctor, medical specialty, female, age 20–30*

> The combination of COVID, increased work pressures, change in environment, and exams together with personal stress can be very challenging.
>
> *Junior doctor, community care, female, age 31–40*

> For half a year our rosters have been non-compliant with College requirements. This has been taken in good faith due to the unprecedented nature of the pandemic, but we're never consulted, never informed of changes until they've been implemented. The result is the overwhelming feeling that we're here for service provision and that our training no longer matters.
>
> *Junior doctor, intensive care, male, age 20–30*

> I really worry about the impact of COVID on trainees. Our registrars are working in our "respiratory zone" with support and supervision available as needed—but not with constant support. We keep hearing comments from them: "I'm the lamb to the slaughter tonight, am I?" and "If a trainee died from COVID would anyone even care?"—which is extremely worrying. I suspect we underestimate the stress they are under.
>
> *Senior doctor, emergency department, female, age 31–40*

As a junior doctor being rotated throughout the pandemic and trying to learn new roles whilst dealing with COVID has made the year more challenging.

Junior doctor, medical specialty, female, age 20–30

We need better workforce planning, rosters in advance, reduced on-call burden, ability to claim for unrostered overtime. The most meaningful intervention you could do for junior doctors is audit the amount of actual overtime they are doing and pay it.

Junior doctor, respiratory medicine, female, age 20–30

Outdated technology

Healthcare workers also wrote about their frustration with the state of technology in the healthcare sector. Reliance on outdated computer systems, faxes, and pagers were especially challenging with the abrupt shift to telehealth. Healthcare workers described the challenges of working remotely with unreliable technology and inadequate network capacity.

COVID-19 has been good in encouraging us to move forward with technology and try different stuff. The downside was this happened so quickly, a lot of us were learning as we went and there weren't yet the resources we needed.

Speech pathologist, community care, female, age 31–40

From a microbiology and infectious disease standpoint, state-of-the-art, high-capacity equipment is needed in labs now. Some machines we currently have are as old as I am, are slow, and have low capacity. Newer machines are faster, have high capacity and can be used remotely, allowing some staff to work from home and lowering the risk of contracting whatever organism is causing a pandemic.

Technician, pathology, male, age 31–40

Some wards and departments still use paper histories, some are computer based. If you are required to work remotely, understanding the patient situation is impossible with paper notes as you have no access.

Social worker, respiratory medicine, female, age 41–50

We spend ridiculous amounts of time in [the state of] Victoria FAXING requests for swab tests done at another hospital because someone has presented at our Emergency Department three days later—and getting the fax hours or days later.

Junior doctor, male, age 31–40

> The pandemic has highlighted the need for equipment and computer upgrades.
>
> *Administrative worker, female, age 51–64*

> With a few things put in place—a computer program to make calls from, VPN access to the server—nurse bank admin staff could have worked from home which would have made all of us feel safer and less anxious.
>
> *Administrative worker, female, age 31–40*

Concerns about fairness and justice

Finally, healthcare workers expressed deep concern about the disproportionate burden of the pandemic on marginalised and vulnerable communities. They were especially concerned about the lack of attention to issues of equity and social justice in pandemic planning and delivery of care. They called for greater inclusion and resources for these cohorts, including Aboriginal and Torres Strait Islander peoples, older adults living in aged care, people with disabilities or mental illness, those living in poverty, and those from culturally and linguistically diverse backgrounds.

> The main challenge was advocating for a pandemic plan for our Aboriginal and Torres Strait Islander community—getting the primary healthcare network to understand the seriousness of the situation.
>
> *General practitioner, female, age 41–50*

> The State and the primary healthcare networks were not talking effectively to our patients in the culturally and linguistically diverse and Aboriginal and Torres Strait Islander Communities. We had to do this ourselves, we had to do our own research, and interpret the guidelines for ourselves.
>
> *General practitioner, male, age 51–64*

> The impact of this pandemic will be felt for many years in the mental health space. So far, no extra funding has made it to public mental health where an already under-funded system is being stretched to breaking point.
>
> *Social worker, community care, female, age 41–50*

> The people who will do worst as a result of the pandemic do worst anyway because of how society is structured. I feel that our health system has placed the welfare of patients second to the welfare of staff and the system.
>
> *Senior doctor, general medicine, male, age 41–50*

> Having experienced this, hopefully we can distribute resources in a more equitable fashion in future. What about poor people and the elderly?
>
> *Nurse, hospital aged care, female, age 51–64*

We need better structures in place to care for geriatric patients. The system is designed to treat this cohort of patients as second-class citizens when they are the most vulnerable.

Junior doctor, hospital aged care, female, age 31–40

There needs to be more support for those in the community that have lost employment, have medical issues, or are living on their own. There is a significant gap in ability for people to access medical care, resulting in very poor patient outcomes.

Paramedic, female, age 20–30

I feel the government overlooked people with a disability as an at-risk group resulting in delayed support.

Disability support worker, community care, female, age 20–30

There needed to be a compassionate approach to culturally and linguistically diverse communities, especially the emergent communities.

General practitioner, female, age 51–64

We must not lose focus of what clients need and how best to meet those needs. We need more translated materials for culturally and linguistically diverse clients.

Nurse, medical specialty, female, age 41–50

We need strong health messaging that targets all members of the community, not just the English-speaking majority.

Junior doctor, anaesthetics, female, age 31–40

13

NOT ABLE TO HUG A DYING PATIENT

> The pandemic and the use of PPE and social distancing has had a huge effect on the interaction between the healthcare worker and patients and relatives. The inability to be able to touch or comfort people has, in my opinion, devalued my reason for working in the palliative care field.
>
> *Nurse, palliative care, female, age 51–64*

The COVID-19 pandemic changed much about the delivery of patient care. Fundamental elements of the process of caring and interacting with patients were disrupted. Social distancing and use of PPE constrained gestures of compassion through touch and facial expressions. Changes to care also meant that healthcare workers were witnesses to, or actors in, events that violated their approach to caring for and treating patients. Healthcare workers described feelings of moral distress as they worried about the effects on care when wearing PPE, barriers to providing timely treatment, the rigidity of visitor restrictions, and care for patients who were dying. In this chapter, healthcare workers describe their experience of grappling with these changes to patient care, emotionally charged interactions with family and patients, and dealing with a public that was at times hostile to healthcare workers who were trying to do their job.

PPE, patients, and care

As we heard in Chapter 7, healthcare workers described many issues associated with PPE. Their concerns included new challenges in patient care, including impaired verbal and non-verbal communication. They noted that obscuring faces with masks was particularly problematic for patients with poor hearing, impaired cognition due to dementia or delirium, or mental health issues such as paranoia or post-traumatic

DOI: 10.4324/9781003228394-13

stress disorder for whom facial expressions and visual cues may be particularly important in communication.

> When patients enter here, all they see is masks.
>
> *Administrative worker, medical specialty, female, 41–50*

> The wearing of masks has made caring for patients so much harder. You can't see their faces and read their expressions which is so important.
>
> *Nurse, emergency department, male, age 51–64*

> PPE is a barrier to care in the mental health field. It can increase mental distress and paranoia and has been associated with triggers of past trauma.
>
> *Occupational therapist, community care, female, age 20–30*

> I worry that I can't deliver the care I want to if I am constantly changing in and out of PPE between a room of a COVID-positive patient and a non-COVID patient.
>
> *Nurse, emergency department, female, age 20–30*

> Constant PPE throughout the whole department does not cause less care to COVID patients so much, but actually causes less time spent with non-COVID patients.
>
> *Nurse, emergency department, female, age 31–40*

> Wearing a mask and face shield around someone with dementia is hard on them as they don't like you wearing them. Also, it's hard for the residents to tell who is who behind the mask.
>
> *Nurse, hospital aged care, female, age 31–40*

> PPE has mainly impacted our area as we are dealing with elderly clients, many of whom have poor or decreased hearing and can't hear people who are wearing masks as they can't read lips or facial expressions.
>
> *Occupational therapist, community care, female, age 41–50*

> It's quite draining working during the pandemic. It saddens me to send family away from being with patients. I have felt very distant wearing PPE. Feels antisocial. Can't see a smile. The residents can't see you smile at them.
>
> *Nurse, hospital aged care, female, age 51–64*

Along with PPE, healthcare workers described other changes that influenced the care they were able to provide to patients. Some of these challenges occurred in the context of the increased complexity of patients presenting for face-to-face treatment, for whom telehealth was not the best option.

> As a clinician I'm seeing more and more people present to the emergency department and when you strip away their "presenting problem" you can see the COVID anxiety, loneliness, fear, and uncertainty. Especially in the elderly who live alone. I feel more should have been done with a real-world approach. All this online, virtual, Zoom, technology stuff just doesn't have the beneficial result of talking to and being with people.
>
> *Nurse, emergency department, male, age 51–64*

> My patients are sicker, with many more mental health presentations. Definitely have adjusted to telehealth, but it remains hard to limit contact with patients: no hugs, no holding newborns unless medically indicated, no unnecessary examination. There's still some grief about losing the rituals of physical contact of our profession.
>
> *General practitioner, female, age 31–40*

> I personally miss treating patients face-to-face. I feel I was good at that. I don't want to lose that as part of my role, it's important. Not everything can be done over telehealth, just because we have access to the technology.
>
> *Occupational therapist, hand therapy, female, age 31–40*

Healthcare workers emphasised the importance of the emotional, as well as clinical, dimensions of care.

> It's more difficult to give my clients the time and connection I want to give or gave before. Lots of procedures, less heart.
>
> *Occupational therapist, community care, female, age 51–64*

> In doing our jobs, we are given a hammer and rivets. We are not able to do our work as intended. We are not caring; we are not treating. We are all fatigued, stressed, and can't breathe. This is so unfair and meaningless.
>
> *Nurse, emergency department, male, age 31–40*

Compromised care

Many healthcare workers felt that the care that they provided was compromised during this period. They talked about the feelings of guilt and moral distress that resulted when they felt unable to provide their usual high standard of care.

> Guilt has been a factor that I didn't expect in dealing with the pandemic. As a health practitioner there is an expectation, and not fulfilling that expectation makes me feel I let people down.
>
> *Nurse, palliative care, female, age 51–64*

The strain of these challenging conditions does affect the quality of care provided by all of the team and it is noticeable.

Nurse, emergency department, female, age 20–30

No amount of "counselling" will support an individual to deal with the burnout and moral injury of not being able to do one's job well, which a lack of resources produces.

Psychologist, community care, female, age 41–50

I think I have been burdened by the feeling that this pandemic has caused a decline in the quality of care we are providing to our patients, for our own safety. Procedures being delayed, families not being allowed to visit.

Nurse, intensive care, female, age 31–40

When caring for a COVID patient over a month ago, I found it extremely confronting that I couldn't care for them as I normally would due to PPE and lack of a clear medical plan. That was draining.

Nurse, surgical, female, age 31–40

Nursing is much less satisfying when we have to be so concerned about patient contact, not allowing patients in clinic for more than so many minutes, and also having to treat patients with a cold as if they have COVID-19.

Nurse, community care, female, age 31–40

I have never had "mental health" issues before. It's very hard as a healthcare worker to accept that you aren't coping and need help. Many health care workers derive self-esteem by doing a good job caring for their patients. When you can't do your job well—due to the pandemic—it causes unexpected stress.

Senior doctor, surgical, female, age 41–50

Moral distress and dying alone

During the pandemic, new rules aimed at preventing the spread of infection changed many aspects of care. Few rules caused as much distress—to patients, their families, and healthcare workers—as the harsh restrictions on visitors. In some facilities, visitors were banned entirely. Elsewhere, one or two family members were able to be present, for limited periods of time, as life was beginning (in the labour wards of maternity hospitals) or ending (for patients in the final days of palliative care). Many patients suffered, and some died, alone. Healthcare workers described the emotional trauma that this separation caused to patients, families, and healthcare workers; and the profound changes to their roles that resulted.

I am devastated our dying patients have been denied open access from family and immediate friends, and funerals are a very lonely experience for some. Interstate family members most often cannot attend due to restrictions. Surely there needs to be more compassion and flexibility? It makes me sick to think these dear people feel alone and families feel helpless.

Nurse, palliative care, female, age 51–64

Keeping people in nursing homes, apart from their families, is such a gross mismanagement and goes totally against the aged care ethos, that I find it totally horrendous trying to comprehend. They are just letting the elderly die of broken hearts—completely alone—and it is inhumane and frightening.

Technician, medical imaging, female, age 51–64

It is a nightmare. I feel as though it's taken everything away from nursing that I love. Holding an iPad to a dying patient to say goodbye and not being able to hug them or care for them like we used to. It's horrible.

Nurse, surgical, female, age 31–40

It's very hard to watch family say goodbye to their loved ones over an iPad. It's a big responsibility to be the intermediary between an unconscious dying patient and their loved ones calling out to them over an iPad. I think this will affect me for a long time.

Nurse, hospital aged care, female, age 41–50

Watching vulnerable older people die without their family able to visit. Emotions from families, especially about patients who contracted COVID in hospital. Having to break bad news, or discuss the pandemic with distraught relatives, multiple times per day. All while trying to care for patients who are deaf and cognitively impaired while in PPE.

Junior doctor, hospital aged care, female, age 20–30

I found that when I had a patient who was palliative, it was extremely difficult when only two visitors were allowed to come and say goodbye. I already struggle with providing support to families, as their loved ones pass, and this made it even harder.

Nurse, medical specialty, female, age 20–30

The hardest part of being a nurse has been caring for lonely people. Providing end-of-life care to people who are unable to have visitors. This has been awful and has led me to cry on the way home on multiple occasions.

Nurse, intensive care, female, age 41–50

Caring for patients dying alone is awful. Managing family distress, and feeling blamed for this, is awful. Careful attention needs to be paid to the impact on non-COVID-19 patients.

Junior doctor, respiratory medicine, female, age 20–30

Seeing the impact of visitor restrictions on patients' palliative care experience is very hard. I feel that the cumulative effect of months of this is really taking its toll on everyone.

Senior doctor, palliative care, female, age 41–50

It isn't just COVID patients who haven't had their loved ones with them at death. It has been an enormous strain on palliative services to keep clients home and out of hospital. The ripple effect is far more widespread than just COVID patients and the hospitals.

Nurse, palliative care, female, age 51–64

A lot of my patients are dying of COVID, as I work for a hospital that does visits to aged care facilities that are hotspots. I am grateful I can be of service to such a vulnerable population, but the effects of the lockdown are devastating for everyone. A large proportion of my day is spent comforting distressed families. This has the biggest impact on me.

Junior doctor, emergency department, female, age 31–40

We need to pay more attention to the wellbeing of nursing home patients. Their families are often their only comfort and denying them visits for extended periods is very cruel. We must also allow patients good deaths and adequate family support during illness, or we risk causing more suffering than even COVID is capable of. The suffering caused by knowing a parent died alone does not end when that parent dies, and I expect the mental health effects of some of our distancing interventions will linger for years.

Senior doctor, medical specialty, female, age 41–50

Visitors

The detrimental consequences of visitor restrictions were felt across all areas of healthcare, not just when patients were dying. Even when they acknowledged that such restrictions were needed, healthcare workers identified manifold harms associated with visitor restrictions. Keeping families informed became an additional responsibility; the dynamics of this communication shifted as families were fearful and frustrated because they couldn't see their loved ones. Overstretched healthcare workers needed to dig deep to find the extra reserves of time and energy required while being called on to act in ways that violated their moral compass.

> Now, every day, I am telling family members they can't visit their loved ones. I am concerned events like this will create irreparable trauma to people on one scale or another. I think that will be another crisis our health care system is not prepared for.
>
> *Administrative worker, medical specialty, female, age 31–40*

> The impacts on health caused by visitor restrictions are not currently being considered adequately and are leading to, currently unmeasured, long-lasting harm.
>
> *Senior doctor, emergency department, male, age 41–50*

> We needed an increase in translator services for culturally and linguistically diverse patients as visitors were not allowed, making communication more difficult.
>
> *Nurse, surgical, female, age 20–30*

Some healthcare workers were grateful that virtual visits through video calls were possible. However, these were generally seen as a poor substitute for having loved ones present at the bedside.

> I am mostly seeing the effect of restrictions on people admitted without COVID. We had one patient recently admitted from the country after a stroke. His wife came down in the ambulance, but was unable to stay with him. Very difficult for the family. We've had many instances like this. I'm very thankful to be working on the virtual visitor program and helping these families out.
>
> *Nurse, hospital-based, female, age 51–64*

> Lack of visitors is devastating for inpatients. Initiatives to facilitate FaceTime conversations with the use of tablets on wards has been invaluable.
>
> *Occupational therapist, hospital aged care, female, age 31–40*

> Telehealth access seemed to help some families when they could see their loved ones in hospital.
>
> *Senior doctor, intensive care, female, age 31–40*

> It's really difficult that people are alone in the hospital, no matter why they are there. Telehealth is helpful, but doesn't replace a physical visitor.
>
> *Nurse, intensive care, female, age 31–40*

Throughout their comments, the emotional impact of visitor restrictions on healthcare workers was clear, as was the increased load that healthcare workers carried providing emotional support to patients and families during these periods of separation.

> Not letting family members see their loved ones has taken a significant toll on me. I cry for those families every day.
>
> *Administrative worker, medical specialty, female, age 31–40*

> Families not allowed to visit patients has been awful.
>
> *Nurse, intensive care, female, age 51–64*

> I've found the most traumatic element of the pandemic has been turning away family and friends of both COVID and non-COVID patients. While the no-visitor policy has been absolutely vital, to promote staff and patient safety, it doesn't make telling a mother she can't visit her son (who has just been in a horrific car accident and is now in a coma) any easier.
>
> *Nurse, intensive care, female, age 20–30*

> No visitors to hospital makes my job far more difficult but it is necessary for patient and staff safety.
>
> *Junior doctor, palliative care, male, age 41–50*

> Because our patients aren't able to have their loved ones around as much, a lot of our patients' emotional support is coming from us. Perhaps more emotional support for patients in hospital would have been beneficial to take some weight off our shoulders.
>
> *Nurse, surgical, female, age 20–30*

> Patients not being able to have visitors means more time spent on the phone updating family, rather than just being able to update patient and family in the room all at one time.
>
> *Junior doctor, emergency department, female, age 20–30*

> The lack of visitors for all our ICU patients has added to the stress and emotional impact. Being the person [that provides all the emotional support] all the time is difficult for critically ill patients, and we sympathise greatly with both the patient and their loved ones through this time.
>
> *Nursing, intensive care, female, age 41–50*

Healthcare workers pointed to the important roles that family and friends play in the care process.

> I hate that patients aren't allowed to have visitors. Especially a lot of the general medicine patients who have cognitive impairments, or are close to end of life without being in the last week of life, or English isn't their first language. Their care and hospital experience would be so much better if they were allowed a visitor to help them understand the treatment plan during

> ward rounds and encourage them to eat at meal times. It would take a lot of pressure off staff.
>
> *Junior doctor, general medicine, female, age 20–30*

> The impersonal nature of the work with patients. In ICU family are usually how we get to know patients that are unconscious. The PPE severely affects our workflow and ability to give proper care.
>
> *Nurse, intensive care, female, age 31–40*

> Lack of allowing carers into the hospital when patients are critically unwell, or for young adolescents who still live with their parents, is distressing for families and for staff. It has an impact on the care we are able to provide as valuable information is missing.
>
> *Senior doctor, emergency department, female, age 41–50*

Midwives wrote about the harm of excluding support people during cardinal life events such as childbirth.

> Midwives are big empaths and restricting a mother's support people is distressing for the mother and her family. Healthcare workers are verbally abused due to this and there has been a lack of support from management acknowledging that this is an issue. Wearing full PPE is stressful, especially when caring for women in labour and trying to support their physical and emotional needs that are exacerbated at this time. Women in labour do not just lay in bed and stay still, they are constantly moving around the room. Top this off with wearing a plastic gown that makes you sweat whilst you are trying to look after and reassure a distressed woman. It is not a pleasant time at work.
>
> *Midwife, female, age 20–30*

> Not having support people on maternity wards is difficult for staff. Patients are emotional and need help looking after their baby if they have had a Caesarean-section. It increases the workload of midwives, sometimes having to do basic care for babies like changing nappies that mums are unable to do, also settling babies on night shift and so on.
>
> *Nurse, maternity, female, age 41–50*

Wider health repercussions

The reduction in services that occurred as a result of lockdown restrictions was significant. Throughout their comments, healthcare workers wrote about the wider repercussions of the pandemic for the health of communities. Two areas of particular concern were worsening of mental health and delayed presentations.

Worsening of mental health

Healthcare workers told us that mental health presentations had increased in both frequency and complexity.

> The patients we are seeing have problems we cannot fix medically in an acute inpatient stay (financial insecurity, family violence, self-harm, overdoses, alcoholism). We have always had these cases but the sheer number of these now is huge, with a corresponding decrease in "easy" cases like pyelonephritis and viral gastroenteritis.
>
> *Senior doctor, general medicine, female, age 31–40*

> My team and I are experiencing an increase in mental health patient caseload: increased client complexity, increased suicidal thoughts and attempts, increased drug use, behavioural problems, aggression, anxiety, and difficult-to-manage behaviour from families.
>
> *Social worker, community care, female, age 31–40*

> In general, I don't feel differently about my work or patients. We have always had to look after patients with complicated infectious diseases in isolation—it's just that now there are greater numbers. I do the best I can, but some patients are coming in with, or acquiring, significant, difficult behaviours that make caring for them hard.
>
> *Nurse, intensive care, female, age 51–64*

> The mental health system is broken and cannot cope with the influx and acuity of patients, both inpatient and community-wise. We are all burning out more rapidly than usual because we cannot provide the support we normally can.
>
> *Occupational therapist, community care, female, age 20–30*

> We've had increased mental health admissions that may have taken more of a toll than the average medical case. Similar situations with elderly patients who have lived alone and are neglecting their own health due to not wanting to leave the house, and therefore turning up to hospital worse and creating stressful and critical situations for nursing and medical staff.
>
> *Nurse, emergency department, female, age 20–30*

> During the lockdown I did notice a marked deterioration in my more vulnerable clients' mental health and an improvement in their presentation after lockdown.
>
> *Psychologist, community care, male, age 51–64*

> The decision to increase [funding for] psychology sessions from 10 to 20 is well-meaning, but the patients who really need them, can't afford the out-of-pocket of $70 plus per visit.
>
> *General practitioner, female, age 51–64*

> My patients are sicker, with many more mental health presentations.
>
> *General practitioner, female, age 31–40*

Delayed presentations

Healthcare workers worried that patients were presenting later in their illness, making their condition more difficult to treat. Sometimes these delayed presentations were due to patients feeling worried about the risk of contracting COVID-19 in hospital. At other times, healthcare workers believed that patients did not want to be a burden on the healthcare system, or simply could not access their usual care provider due to practice closures or travel restrictions.

> My mother, who lives with us, has a recurrent bowel cancer diagnosis. Under normal circumstances she probably could have commenced chemotherapy, but now she is not able to be offered treatment. We just wait, watch, and act if symptoms arise.
>
> *Administrative worker, surgical, female, age 51–64*

> Major concern that patients with potentially curable cancers are not presenting.
>
> *Senior doctor, surgical, male, age 51–64*

> I am aware of a patient with a severe adverse outcome (death) that can be directly attributed to the reduction in community resources available to a family that has occurred as a result of COVID.
>
> *Senior doctor, intensive care, female, age 51–64*

> The hardest thing was drawing up protocols of how we would wind back, and potentially stop, chemotherapy treatments on our patients if the pandemic was to become overwhelming.
>
> *Senior doctor, medical specialty, male, age 51–64*

> I have been concerned that some patients are not seeking care during COVID-19, because they are afraid to come to hospital. Also concerned that whilst telehealth is very useful, it can sometimes give a false sense of assessing or seeing patients, when really, they need to be assessed face to face.
>
> *Physiotherapist, respiratory medicine, female, age 41–50*

Border closures, and denial of border passes, are appalling and are having a severe effect on communities and individuals. Emergency services have been denied access to cross state borders on some occasions due to inappropriate restrictions in place.

Paramedic, female, age 20–30

So much general anxiety about people not accessing regular healthcare and the lack of presentations to hospital. The health system may not cope with the bounceback after we ease the restrictions.

Student, surgical, female, age 20–30

I feel that other health concerns are not seen as a priority. Hospitals are only concerned with COVID. There are other health conditions that are making us unwell, and unless it is COVID, it is hard to get treatment.

Dental assistant, community care, female, age 41–50

We have received referrals for patients who need help and have been directed to not visit them unless they are a category one [urgent] patient. It is very hard to engage with elderly and vulnerable patients over the phone. You feel guilty that you can't serve these patients as you normally would, and yet the hospital holds you responsible if something goes wrong.

Nurse, community care, female, age 41–50

My usual service, continence, was closed leaving many vulnerable people in the community without assistance which has caused significant stress for them—and me—as referrals keep piling up and we are unable to attend to them.

Nurse, community care, female, age 51–64

I feel that many patients didn't receive the care they required, or delayed care, as patients were not able to have aerosol-generating procedures in general wards, due to not having negative pressure rooms.

Nurse, intensive care, male, age 31–40

I have been concerned that some patients are not seeking care during COVID-19, because they are afraid to come to hospital.

Physiotherapist, respiratory medicine, female, age 41–50

Observations in working with surgeons is they are concerned that people could be at a disadvantage with their health and not presenting with potentially life-threatening issues because of COVID keeping them away from hospitals. Also, theatre lists reduced, leaving waiting-lists to grow and more people having to wait and suffer.

Administrative worker, surgical, female, age 51–64

> The longer this goes on, the more I am worried about the impact on patients waiting to have procedures done for conditions that impact their livelihoods and quality of life.
>
> *Senior doctor, surgical, male, age 51–64*

Bearing the brunt of patient and family distress

Profound changes to care delivery, restrictions on visitors, and anxiety among patients and the community proved to be an explosive mix, with emotions running high in many interactions with patients and families. Healthcare workers told us that rates of verbal, and sometimes physical, aggression worsened during the pandemic, as people's frustrations and fears spilled over onto those doing their best to provide care in difficult circumstances.

> Code Greys and Code Blacks [emergency codes used in hospitals to alert security to threatening behaviour and aggression] for violence are up something like 80 percent in the emergency department I work in alone.
>
> *Nurse, emergency department, female, age 20–30*

> This has caused increased assaults on the ward and a general sense of fear amongst staff.
>
> *Occupational therapist, community care, female, age 20–30*

> Educating patients to go get tested for COVID is crucial. They are coming in for cough syrup, and when asked if they have had a COVID test they get angry for even getting asked.
>
> *Pharmacist, female, age 20–30*

> Families and some patients tend to take it out on nursing staff. Patients are wanting everything now, but donning PPE takes time and a lot of them don't really understand. Families tend to abuse staff on the phone. You try your best initially but it's just more exhausting.
>
> *Nurse, hospital aged care, female, age 51–64*

> All the children in outpatients have high levels of anxiety, challenging behaviours, or other mental health symptoms and our service is not equipped to offer any psychology. Private psychology services cannot be afforded by most families and they have long waiting-lists at present. This has made my outpatient work frustrating, and not rewarding, due to my inability to assist these families and children. Families often transmit their frustration onto me which is straining! We need to bring psychology into schools or have better access through the public health system.
>
> *Senior doctor, paediatrics, female, age 31–40*

The hardest challenge has been the verbal abuse of nurses—over the phone from families—and nurses not feeling like they could hang up, so experiencing aggression silently. Nurses from the hospital, going to save residential aged care residents, and being yelled at and abused by families at the front door and carpark.

Nurse, hospital-based, female, age 41–50

While doing a COVID test on a patient, I was punched in the jaw by a patient because they found the test unpleasant.

Nurse, emergency department, female, age 20–30

I'm working as an advanced trainee in an inpatient palliative care unit with harsh visitor restrictions (no-one is allowed in or out unless "very end of life"). The levels of distress and anger from patients and families are so high. I know people are so upset and scared, but it's a lot to manage when you're bearing the brunt of it all day.

Junior doctor, palliative care, female, age 20–30

Regarding hospital pharmacy, medicines shortages have continued to be an issue throughout the pandemic for short periods of time due to supply chain shortages. This has put extra strain on the pharmacist-patient relationship. Sometimes patients don't understand when the exact brand of medicine, or type of medicine they want, is currently not in stock. Most patients are understanding, but on top of the other COVID issues in the hospital when a patient snaps at you it can be disheartening.

Pharmacist, hospital aged care, male, age 20–30

Provide greater education to the community regarding current hospital policy and procedures during a pandemic. This would reduce abuse towards staff therefore increasing mental health. At the moment I feel we keep on getting kicked down and not a lot of good is coming to us. We can only keep getting kicked down so many times.

Nurse, emergency department, female, age 31–40

14

SUPPORTING EMOTIONAL WELLBEING

> Asking for supports and help is difficult for some in terms of lack of time, worry about stigma, or difficulty disclosing feelings.
>
> *General practitioner, female, age 51–64*

Healthcare workers are a precious resource in the public health response to COVID-19. However, as we have heard in previous chapters, they need workplace support as they struggle with the demands of providing care during the pandemic. In this chapter healthcare workers describe the struggles they face in seeking support for mental health, what they perceive as helpful, and what they believe would help in supporting them into the future. Healthcare workers emphasised the importance of shifting the responsibility for workplace health and wellbeing away from the individual, by embedding supportive strategies into healthcare systems and institutions.

Obstacles to seeking support

Only a minority of respondents reported that they had accessed professional services for emotional wellbeing or mental health distress. Some wrote about the reluctance of healthcare workers to seek help.

> As health care workers we are often very bad at looking after ourselves. Ironic.
>
> *Respiratory scientist, male, age 51–64*

> I think that there hasn't been much attention paid to the emotional wellbeing of healthcare workers—especially those juggling multiple responsibilities outside of work and those that are geographically isolated from loved

DOI: 10.4324/9781003228394-14

ones. Every day I see a colleague struggling—and not many are seeking help from the workplace.

Physiotherapist, intensive care, female, age 31–40

I was reluctant to seek help, as I never had before. It was unclear the first step to take.

Senior doctor, emergency department, male, age 51–64

Culture and stigma

They gave several reasons why healthcare workers might be reluctant to access help and support. One reason was an entrenched culture of suffering in silence, linked to internalised and professional stigma around help-seeking for mental illness.

Most health professionals try to intellectualise problems and cope and feel guilty about asking for help. There needs to be a cultural shift in medicine, and not just because of the pandemic.

Senior doctor, medical specialty, female, age 31–40

Try to make counselling sessions a mandatory monthly appointment for health care workers. Particularly those that have had NO changes to their rosters and worked all through the pandemic to date. Don't wait for them to ask, they are not likely the ones to ask for some mental health days—they will suffer in silence until they break.

Dental assistant, surgical, female, age 51–64

Most hospitals have tried to provide avenues of supports, but I think many of us aren't used to using them. And it seems like yet another thing to do. Forums are offered but how to find time on top of our usual work.

Senior doctor, surgical, female, age 41–50

Some healthcare workers wrote about the invalidating responses of managers and other leaders if they shared their emotional struggles or their need to access professional supports.

If I tried to speak up, I was told that "other people have also had to suffer" and to "get on with it". I am very happy to work hard and pride myself on it actually, but there was no space to speak up and say it has been a struggle.

Junior doctor, intensive care, female, age 31–40

There is a pre-existing culture, in the health service I work in, that if an employee discloses mental health issues they are seen as a liability. The "support" available to employees is conditional. The risk of being bullied out

> of the health service if you disclose a mental health issue has exponentially increased since the pandemic.
>
> *Physiotherapist, hospital outpatients, female, age 41–50*

> Not all those in supposed leadership roles show empathy or support. Some are like "just get on with it". This is very disturbing, this is what led to my anxieties!
>
> *Nurse, hospital aged care, female, age 41–50*

> You had to adapt regardless of how you were feeling. If you said you "needed a minute" to have a breath because you were feeling overcome with anxiety, you were told to "suck it up".
>
> *Nurse, medical specialty, female, age 20–30*

> There is still stigma and guilt around mental health, especially in country areas where it is seen as a weakness and letting the team down. The supports are in place, but, although I have sought help, I don't openly talk about it. I use a physical ailment to cover for my mental health issues.
>
> *Nurse, perioperative care, female, age 41–50*

Privacy and confidentiality

Reluctance to seek support was also linked to fears about privacy and confidentiality, especially if accessing support through their workplace.

> I would like to seek some brief psychological help, but I have been working in my local area for so long, it's hard to find somebody who does not know me.
>
> *General practitioner, female, age 65–70*

> I don't want to see my GP about how I'm feeling as she refers patients to me!
>
> *Senior doctor, medical specialty, female, age 41–50*

> Nurses are afraid to disclose if they are having difficulty coping or are anxious or depressed. Workplaces overreact and start notifying insurers if a nurse discloses that the workplace is causing stress or anxiety.
>
> *Nurse, community care, female, age 31–40*

Concern about confidentiality was one reason for reluctance to use professional supports linked to their workplaces such as Employee Assistance Programs (EAP).

> I have been reluctant to talk to EAP due to confidentiality issues.
>
> *Social worker, medical specialty, female, age 51–64*

> EAP is not "free" or "confidential". It is billed to a cost-centre, which your line-manager can see, in the health service I work in. Your name and the number of sessions you have accessed is disclosed to your line-manager. Some staff do not access EAP for this very reason.
>
> *Physiotherapist, hospital outpatients, female, age 41–50*

> I have had significant impacts on my wellbeing, for numerous reasons, and I am predisposed to anxiety and depression. I am working on my own wellbeing plan. However, I will not approach my workplace for EAP as you have to see a GP in staff care to access it. I have voiced numerous times that this is inappropriate—but it falls on deaf ears. I am happy that there are other services I can turn to [outside of my workplace] if my wellbeing doesn't improve for advice. I also feel as though we have a good culture in our consultant group and I could contact a peer for advice too.
>
> *Senior doctor, emergency department, female, age 31–40*

Time and energy

Difficulty finding the time and energy to access services when needed was mentioned by many.

> More supports during work hours would be helpful. Although there's EAP and other supports to access after work, by the time you finish for the day it can be too tiring to want to speak to anyone.
>
> *Allied health practitioner, community mental health, female, age 31–40*

> I have been reluctant to contact EAP as I'm so busy at work and I want to try to forget it when I get home. Allocated time or an increased focus at work may encourage people to seek assistance.
>
> *Nurse, medical specialty, female, age 51–64*

> Even if I chose to seek help, I simply don't have enough time to do anything about it.
>
> *Medical scientist, medical specialty, female, age 51–64*

> My colleagues and I are emotionally drained. While I know there are supports in place they are not advertised very clearly, and people seem too tired to reach out for help.
>
> *Nurse, general medicine, female, age 31–40*

> Often supports are put in place during the day when lots of frontline workers can't access them, such as those in clinic or theatre.
>
> *Junior doctor, anaesthetics, female, age 31–40*

> I think I should talk to a professional, but part of me feels scared, or feels I have no time to do so. And I feel I cannot take a mental health day as we are short on staff; that'd make me feel irresponsible if I took a day off.
>
> *Junior doctor, emergency department, female, age 20–30*

> Resources can be great, however regardless of the quality of the resource, nurses need the space and time to be able to utilise them. Having more nurses on shift would give them the space to be able to take time away from the clinical space. Short term this may be difficult, but investing in nurses for the long-term is of greater benefit to the industry as a whole.
>
> *Nurse, intensive care, female, age 31–40*

> There is actually so much stuff about wellbeing crossing my desk. I don't read it. So it's not that I don't know the opportunity is there, I just can't muster the energy to do yet more things!
>
> *Senior doctor, palliative care, female, age 41–50*

Existing supports that were helpful

Healthcare workers were appreciative when team leaders, managers, and other colleagues showed that they cared by regularly checking in with them about how they were coping.

> Regular contact from our medical director and support teams has helped me through the pandemic and personal illness.
>
> *Junior doctor, community care, female, age 31–40*

> Our staff in the emergency department were at the forefront of welfare checking for staff within the department. They set up a system of check-ins and welfare deliveries etc. They didn't rely on management for doing this. All the emails in the world about the EAP weren't as useful as reaching out with human contact—by phone or doorstop deliveries—to tell people we were thinking about them in their quarantine.
>
> *Nurse, emergency department, female, age 51–64*

Others spoke positively about their experience of using phone lines and other wellbeing resources established by their health service or another professional organisation.

> Being a rural nurse, I have access to the Bush Crisis Line, a service for all rural and remote healthcare workers. Having never contacted a crisis line in my entire life, let alone my rural nursing career, I contacted them twice during this COVID-19 pandemic and found the support absolutely wonderful. This

focused "de-briefing" and "re-framing", and "being-with" made an absolute world of difference to me, my family, and my many patients.

Nurse, community care, male, age 51–64

The best thing at my hospital has been a positive and tireless response from the CEO and the psychology department who have provided extra supports, weekly online psychological wellbeing sessions for staff, tip sheets, and helplines. It's been amazing.

Senior doctor, medical specialty, male, age 51–64

Employer-provided counselling programs were helpful for some, especially if they were easily accessible at work.

Access to EAP has helped me to cope with my increased anxieties and stresses.

Nurse, community care, female, age 41–50

My workplace has brought EAP into the unit. Whilst accessing EAP was always an option, having them physically or virtually in the unit to discuss things privately or with colleagues was a great initiative.

Nurse, intensive care, female, age 31–40

Some healthcare workers accessed professional support outside of their workplaces. Examples included talking to their general practitioner, counsellor, or psychologist.

My GP gave me permission to take time off from work after I had recovered from COVID. I did not understand the emotional toll that having COVID would take on me even though I was not unwell. I was very angry and traumatised when I returned to work. A return to work plan and emotional support via my public health employer would have been good.

Senior doctor, surgical, female, age 41–50

Regular appointments with my psychologist have been a godsend. I would not have been able to make it through the pandemic without these. I am grateful that the government increased the number of sessions that I can use my mental health care plan as this reduces the financial burden of these.

Speech pathologist, medical specialty, female, age 41–50

My psychologist saved my life this year. I was so worried about having a mental health care plan on my record that I waited too long, until it had become a mountain rather than a hill.

Physiotherapist, surgical, female, age 20–30

> Without my psychiatrist's support I think I would not be here, and I have never considered that before.
>
> *Nurse, pathology, female, age 51–64*

More than "one-size-fits-all"

Healthcare workers told us that there was no single "all-purpose" way of providing the support they needed. They advocated for a range of strategies to support healthcare workers in the workplace and also emphasised that support must be responsive to each person's situation and needs.

> It's important to remember that we are a diverse group—there is no one size fits all.
>
> *Senior doctor, palliative care, female, age 51–64*

> We need more than talk. More than impersonal catch-all solutions. Wellbeing solutions that are tailored to the team they are being rolled out to.
>
> *Nurse, general medicine, female, age 31–40*

> Everyone will respond and cope differently, so it's really hard to provide a "one-size-fits-all" solution. I think asking the groups you're trying to support what might help them (and now's a good time to ask because we're in the thick of it)—and interpreting the non-responses as well—to direct what will help. I also think personalized responses help (not a message to all nurses but distributed in more personalized groups). Extroverts want people (this is me, I love community and sharing with others), and I imagine introverts want private reflection, but probably to know there is someone close who cares. It's important to have a big safety net (e.g. employee support phoneline), but also to have a person to talk to if needed.
>
> *Junior doctor, respiratory medicine, female, age 20–30*

> Everyone is different. During furlough there have been thoughtful suggestions to link with peers who are also furloughed, but this was not something that would be helpful for myself.
>
> *Occupational therapist, medical specialty, female, age 31–40*

> People being overly supportive can be just as exhausting as no support! This is just another risk we take, and focusing on the good parts as well as the difficulties is more useful for mental health than focusing solely on how much everyone is struggling. We have had it a lot better than many of our colleagues.
>
> *Junior doctor, general medicine, female, age 20–30*

> I am by nature quite pragmatic and find a lot of the tools available for support not very useful. However, I do know that a friend found them extremely useful which shows that one size does not fit all.
>
> *Nurse, research institute, female, age 51–64*

> People are different and therefore it is important not to assume all people require comfort, or constant debriefing. I have sometimes felt suffocated by too much support, as I will ask when I need it, and I will choose whom I need it from.
>
> *Allied health practitioner, hospital aged care, female, age 41–50*

> All wellbeing is aimed at looking after doctors-in-training. There needs to be care for senior staff, consultants etc even in non-pandemic times. The stresses are huge for senior decision-makers and they need support too.
>
> *Senior doctor, emergency department, female, age 51–64*

Supports that would be helpful

Healthcare workers expressed diverse views on the best way for wellbeing support to be delivered.

Embedding supports into the workplace

Many wrote about the importance of access to on-site debriefing and professional psychologists or therapists, rather than wellbeing apps and other digital or phone resources.

> There was an underestimation of the emotional impact this would have on staff directly working in the thick of the pandemic. Hospitals need more than EAP and care packages. Professional external psychologists should be on site for staff to access professional help.
>
> *Nurse, general medicine, female, age 41–50*

> Having independent mental health workers available for employees to see on-site when needed is crucial. These mental health workers would need to not be employed by the health service.
>
> *Physiotherapist, hospital outpatients, female, age 41–50*

> Phone numbers and services are great, but most people would not pick up the phone to ask for help. If an external person was there, and able to provide confidential support at work, access to mental health care might be improved.
>
> *Pharmacist, general medicine, female, age 31–40*

> I cannot stress enough how much I think nurses would benefit from a mandatory debrief session. It would be great if we could have a good vent and learn some strategies that directly relate to our issues.
>
> *Nurse, residential aged care, female, age 41–50*

> Encourage more people to get therapy—those mindfulness apps aren't a substitute for therapy.
>
> *Nurse, medical imaging, female, age 31–40*

> Personally, I have not found apps helpful, preferring a human face to help. I feel that all healthcare workers are struggling at present as we are damned if we do (in protecting the community) and damned if we don't (limiting visitors to reduce the spread of COVID). But we are NOT OK!
>
> *Nurse, palliative care, female, age 51–64*

> An ICU psychologist for staff and patients would be a valuable addition to any ICU team.
>
> *Nurse, intensive care, female, age 41–50*

> Work sent us to a supposedly "welfare group meeting" which I found did the opposite. It was not well run and did not use a proper psychologist which I thought didn't help with dealing with anxiety but exacerbated it. Hospitals should be using only properly trained welfare officers with a clinical psychology background.
>
> *Senior doctor, anaesthetics, female, age 41–50*

Healthcare workers—particularly those working with COVID-positive patients—thought it would be useful to provide onsite support by way of debriefing sessions and monitoring of fatigue.

> Even small things like a structured "decompression session" at the end of a shift would help.
>
> *Junior doctor, emergency department, female, age 31–40*

> If we look at what the defence forces do after high tempo periods—there is often a "decompression" period where people are mandated to take two weeks off work in the immediate period on returning from a war zone. It is incredibly important we use the period of having extra staff employed on temporary contracts to maximise leave planning for permanent staff.
>
> *Nurse, intensive care, female, age 31–40*

> Fatigue scoring and management should be standard practice in medicine, similar to other industries that are high risk for harming oneself or others such as mining, aviation, and armed forces. I strongly believe that more

appropriate fatigue monitoring and physical health monitoring also would go a long way to improving mental health.

Senior doctor, anaesthetics, female, age 31–40

Outsourcing supports feels impersonal, bringing supports in house and having a "drop in" centre for support would be good. I am in spiritual care and have been offering a lot of impromptu support for staff across the days. I can see this is directly valued and is also indirectly valuable to the teams, the organisation and also patients, of course. Offering regular, non-clinical well-being support (designated in direct response to pandemic), such as spiritual care, available in a central location, onsite for everyone, would be a good idea and very protective.

Allied health practitioner, pastoral care, female, age 41–50

Structured paid professional debriefing is needed for everyone during and after this trauma. Not just emergency departments, intensive care units and psychology. Aged care is often forgotten but we have a very high emotional toll from caring for very vulnerable patients with high mortality rates and high emotions from their families that is understandable and unrelenting. As a registrar I am there on the ground every day and take the brunt of this as the most senior available person. I see the distress of my colleagues and we end up being each other's counsellors when we have little reserves left. I think we would all benefit from having to debrief formally, but we don't have time to do it and see the EAP or formal counselling as something you can only afford to do at the absolute end of the line. It is not accessible unless you take time off, and most of us find it too hard to arrange that or have no option to.

Junior doctor, hospital aged care, female, age 20–30

Safe and supportive working conditions

Many healthcare workers emphasised the need for workplaces to address the underlying conditions causing stress, rather than focusing only on individual support solutions. Suggestions included providing safe physical workspaces, filling gaps in rosters, and scheduling sufficient time for breaks.

The focus should be on addressing the systemic issues that contribute to decreased wellbeing among healthcare workers, rather than perpetuating an individualistic approach of the healthcare workers being responsible for maintaining their own well-being.

Nurse, community care, male, age 20–30

We need actual structured mental health and wellbeing activities. Being told by management that we need to watch our mental health, and them throwing a pizza party, is the equivalent of throwing a Band-Aid over a haemorrhaging artery.

Nurse, emergency department, male, age 20–30

Tokenistic supports (e.g., breakout rooms/yoga sessions) are unhelpful when the workload means you can't access them. Sometimes we barely get a lunch break, where is the time for yoga?

Junior doctor, emergency department, female, age 20–30

It's all good and well to say "meditate, do yoga, and call the Employee Assistance Program". But if there's no ability for you to self-manage your work—the main source of stress—I don't see that the other things can fix that.

Junior doctor, hospital aged care, female, age 20–30

More needs to be done to look after people as a whole—physically, mentally, and emotionally. Making sure we are hydrated, well fed, feel appreciated, and have opportunities to rest.

Junior doctor, emergency department, female, age 31–40

I wish that physical wellbeing during work was taken seriously. I don't need virtual yoga or coffee vouchers—basics like easy access to drinking water, proper breaks, and access to a toilet would be great!

Senior doctor, emergency department, male, age 41–50

I am working at 70 percent of my usual capacity and energy—sometimes less—and I'm usually a high energy person. I observe others in the same boat. Understanding this, and accommodating for it in the work and resourcing, is critical to supporting frontline workers in these situations. It's practical resources like ensuring everyone has a drink and a five-minute break at least hourly in a busy shift when wearing full PPE, that the equipment is available and working, and that you aren't always rostered to the COVID-positive areas or patients.

Nurse, emergency department, female, age 51–64

Stop thinking apps replace humans. They don't.

Allied health practitioner, community outreach, female, age 51–64

More face-to-face support, not just lip service.

Nurse, hospital aged care, female, age 51–64

There are far too many half-hearted and generic recommendations for maintaining wellbeing, such as an app and meditation recommendation. We need more humanistic and interpersonal initiatives within the team and community.

Junior doctor, medical specialty, male, age 31–40

> Most of the self-care advice out there really does not understand the nuances and difficulties of actually working on the front line with COVID-19 patients. General self-care advice, such as "Take a break!" "Take some time off!" "Do something nice for yourself on your lunchbreak!" is super-condescending and completely misses the mark. These are simply not things that frontline workers can do if they stay in their roles. Advice and help that actually takes into account what a frontline health role looks like would be helpful, rather than generic advice for the general population or for non-COVID times.
>
> *Psychologist, infectious diseases, female, age 20–30*

> I appreciate the resources we receive. However, I think that prevention is better than a "cure" and addressing issues such as technology and physical space to do our job would go a long way in reducing the stress and allow us to focus on problem-solving bigger picture things like how we provide the most effective patient care.
>
> *Occupational therapist, community care, female, age 20–30*

> Physical health is critical for mental health. We can have as many little chatty exercises or Zoom meetings as we want, they do not help the core of the problem. We need our physical health.
>
> *Junior doctor, general medicine, male, age 31–40*

> Having supports in place is less relevant than making sure health care workers don't work longer than their capacity to manage the stress. Healthcare workers need adequate time away from work rather than being overworked and told "there is an employee assistance program to help if you are not managing".
>
> *Senior doctor, respiratory medicine, male, age 41–50*

> Having a clear plan at work and well-organised structure, was the best antidote to stress.
>
> *Senior doctor, respiratory medicine, female, age 51–64*

> Assistance needs to be meaningful not tokenistic. My current workplace in the disability sector has shown more real care for me in the last two weeks than the hospital system did in the whole duration of COVID. The offers are REAL, not just done to satisfy a checklist.
>
> *Physiotherapist, surgical, female, age 20–30*

Healthcare workers told us that psychological supports should be offered proactively in their workplaces, instead of waiting for healthcare workers to reach a point of crisis.

> Sometimes it helps if support is simply provided. Don't wait for us to ask.
>
> *Nurse, medical specialty, female, age 20–30*

Coping skills and maintaining mental wellbeing—and where and when to get help and support—should be part of education programs for all staff that work in hospitals. Clinical and non-clinical. Managers and all staff should encourage mental health days and other things that can alleviate stress in workers that may be fatigued or at risk of burnout.

Administrative worker, non-clinical, female, age 41–50

It would be helpful if there were more psychological resources available through work.

Nurse, community care, female, age 31–40

Ensure that the smaller teams are being checked on and supported.

Respiratory scientist, female, age 20–30

Identify health care workers who live alone—who will be isolated from friends and family for prolonged periods of time—and consider what can organisations do to support them.

Paramedic, female, age 31–40

You need to check in on people frequently. The people who are down varies from day to day.

Orthoptist, female, age 51–64

Our organisation didn't do anything about staff wellbeing until six months in … not good enough.

Nurse, medical specialty, female, age 31–40

I wish my employer offered more services to us, sooner, then what they did.

Nurse, hospital aged care, female, age 31–40

It's tricky for bosses to have time to check up on their staff working at home, just for a chat to see how they are going. I think it took three months for a boss to ring me … that's not good.

Administrative worker, non-clinical, female, age 41–50

It would be good to have enforced breaks as well as mandatory protected time to talk with someone—a counsellor or psychologist provided by the hospital.

Nurse, medical specialty, female, age 31–40

Normalising help-seeking

Healthcare workers spoke about the need for change within the culture of healthcare and for efforts to be made to normalise help-seeking and feelings of vulnerability.

I think more communication or resources that normalises the message that "it's ok to feel exhausted/depleted/fatigued/angry" would be helpful. A big part of my journey especially in the early part of the pandemic was realising that everyone was not doing as well as perhaps they wanted everyone to think. When we started being honest with each other it was a big help and opened the doors for more peer-to-peer support to happen.

Nurse, education, female, age 31–40

Getting doctors to look after themselves is hard. Changing culture takes time. Senior staff role-modeling this can be very powerful.

Senior doctor, intensive care, male, age 41–50

It is important to recognise the difficulty with which doctors engage with help. The tick box approach of providing the numbers to psychologists, Lifeline and the EAP is useless. We need to provide private, confidential, discreet access to doctors that are empathic and experienced in dealing with doctors and who will manage the problem appropriately rather than apply a Band-Aid.

Senior doctor, anaesthetics, female, age 51–64

I believe that anonymous counselling might be helpful for health professionals that otherwise might not engage in it. For example, via phone calls or messaging.

Junior doctor, emergency department, female, age 20–30

We need more information on getting confidential help, particularly outside of the organisation.

Nurse, medical specialty, female, age 51–64

Our organisation has been really focused on ensuring the mental health of its staff. This has involved regular email updates from the CEO, staff pizza nights, free food for staff, being encouraged to use the employee assistance program, being encouraged to take annual leave if needed, having senior staff be open about the difficulties they are facing and being understanding that all staff, from cleaning staff to surgeons are having a tough time.

Social worker, community care, female, age 31–40

Having an open discussion with management and opening up about the struggles everyone is facing helped with knowing it's normal to be having a tough time at the moment.

Physiotherapist, medical specialty, male, age 20–30

I think senior nurses need to be more vocal about not being OK. This pandemic is not something any of us have done before. It's OK to cry. It's OK to ask for help.

Nurse, infectious diseases, female, age 31–40

> Knowing that I am not one of the few suffering, but more part of the majority of how health care workers are experiencing [the pandemic] makes me feel less alone and less "defective" as a doctor. The stigma and negative consequences of reaching out for help should be abolished so we do not have to suffer alone and suffer without formal help and support.
>
> *Senior doctor, community care, female, age 41–50*

> We need a change in the culture of healthcare to put more of a focus on taking care of yourself, so you can take care of others, rather than powering through and burning yourself out trying to do it all when you're struggling.
>
> *Speech pathologist, community care, female, age 20–30*

> Supporting wellbeing while not calling out common feelings could be done better. Asking staff to self-recognise burnout is so challenging. Perhaps acknowledging it is normal.
>
> *Nurse, emergency department, female, age 31–40*

> It's OK share your vulnerabilities and admit you're not coping. Stop being a superhero.
>
> *Nurse, community care, female, age 41–50*

The importance of peer support

Other healthcare workers wrote about the value of providing and receiving support from peers. This could occur informally, or through a peer support network such as Hand-n-Hand.

> We have introduced a buddy system at work which helps me focus on others.
>
> *Administrative worker, non-clinical, female, age 51–64*

> I have linked in with Hand-n-Hand as a peer supporter. I have been in contact with Twitter friends that are like-minded to know I'm not in this alone.
>
> *Nurse, emergency department, female, age 31–40*

> With respect, counselling services provide generic advice on looking after yourself. They are not in there with you.
>
> *Nurse, respiratory medicine, female, age 51–64*

> We need the support of colleagues. Peer support programs.
>
> *Senior doctor, emergency department, female, age 41–50*

> In our region, we are trialing a peer-to-peer wellbeing buddy system, where people are matched at their level with a buddy and they check in on each other's wellbeing each week.
>
> *Senior doctor, emergency department, female, age 31–40*

General practice can be a very lonely job. The GP has to take charge to ask for supports and help which might be difficult for some GPs in terms of lack of time, worry or difficulty disclosing feelings. A buddy system would be good.

General practitioner, female, age 51–64

Support sessions are great—smaller team-based sessions are best so as not to feel intimidated to talk up.

Physiotherapist, medical specialty, female, age 31–40

Maybe a peer-peer support group app would be beneficial for any future pandemic? So that staff can really connect with each other at a more personal level.

Nurse, casual pool, female, age 31–40

Nurses never ask for help. So the approach would need to be different than offering help to them. Something casual and relaxed like tea and cake and chats should be organised so it's less in your face than a random formal debrief session. And that it's not rushed, and there's a format to the chats and a facilitator that is also relaxed, sitting down at our level that talks about the stressors on the ward.

Nurse, community care, female, age 20–30

I think perhaps having specific buddies to follow-up would be beneficial. If people are just given the option to reach out for help, often they will not.

Nurse, emergency department, female, age 41–50

I urge everyone involved to at least use one or more of the wellbeing tools to self-evaluate the mental health impact of the pandemic and also to have a support group outside of the work to discuss the mental health impact.

Senior doctor, emergency department, male, age 41–50

15

PURPOSE, COMPASSION, AND GRATITUDE

> Helping people in their greatest time of need is a great gift you give them and yourself. It is very satisfying and rewarding. I find myself in dangerous and infectious situations at times, and I'll keep doing it.
>
> *Paramedic, male, age 41–50*

Despite all the challenges and exhaustion and frustration expressed by healthcare workers, their stories were bound by a collective sense of hope. From ward clerks to social workers to pathologists, many healthcare workers were profoundly grateful for the opportunity to serve their communities. They went into healthcare to help others, and many found a renewed sense of purpose and meaning in the work they did during the pandemic. This chapter shares the insights and wisdom of healthcare workers who sought and found ways to live well in a world turned upside down. These people entered healthcare to be of service to others and drew strength from that sense of purpose. This chapter reveals what it means to be not a hero, but a healer.

Compassion

Healthcare workers talked about the importance of kindness, empathy, support, and compassion to themselves and towards others.

> Be kind to each other.
>
> *Nurse, respiratory medicine, male, age 31–40*

> Maintaining a conversation about the impact of the pandemic as we live through these unique times, I think, is the key to support each other.
>
> *Senior doctor, medical specialty, female, age 51–64*

DOI: 10.4324/9781003228394-15

> We need to change from inside us, let us all be more caring and kinder to each other be it at home or at work. Let's practice empathy all the time.
>
> *General practitioner, general medicine, female, age 51–64*

> Best to stay positive do your bit and support those around you. But I never want to hear the word unprecedented again.
>
> *Nurse, radiology, female, age 51–64*

> The colleagues at work are equally important in one's wellbeing, as much as the family is once we get home. If your colleagues also care about each other at work—no matter how difficult it is—you know you'll get through every day.
>
> *Nurse, general medicine, female, age 41–50*

> Maintain a sense of humour and compassion for others. Look after those who will look after you.
>
> *Senior doctor, anaesthetics, male, age 51–64*

> Knowing that there are groups like the Pandemic Kindness group advocating for and caring about us is immeasurably reassuring.
>
> *Senior doctor, medical specialty, female, age 51–64*

> Realise that colleagues are also stressed and don't take their anger and frustrations on board.
>
> *Nurse, community care female, age 41–50*

> Our overall focus on dealing with staff throughout this pandemic has been on forgiveness and patience. We have tried to portray the message to staff that you don't know what someone else is going through at any particular time, so lead with kindness.
>
> *Nurse, surgical, male, age 41–50*

Healthcare workers believed that cultures of compassion and kindness should be fostered and that altruism was important.

> It will be very helpful if a happy and motivated environment is maintained in the hospital, with colleagues helping each other through these tough times.
>
> *General practitioner, general medicine, female, age 20–30*

> We need to promote a culture of genuine compassion and kindness and validate a sense of vulnerability.
>
> *Psychologist, medical specialty, female, age 41–50*

> We need to build interpersonal skills in our communities, so people are less introspective in their thinking and more empathetic to others. Mateship needs to come back.
>
> *Podiatry, community care, female, age 31–40*

> During this time people should be more united, and focused on how we can help and protect each other holistically, and not just from the virus. It is disheartening that sometimes workers are too focused on their own safety and that they forget about how others are feeling.
>
> *Nurse, medical specialty, female, age 31–40*

Contribution

The pandemic also reinforced healthcare workers' sense of purpose and reasons for entering a healing profession.

> Our primary vocation is caring for sick patients.
>
> *Senior doctor, surgical, male, age 51–64*

> Pharmacists are open to care for others during times of need, often putting others' needs before ours or our families.
>
> *Pharmacist, community care, female, age 31–40*

> When the virus first appeared in Wuhan and the Chinese built a hospital in days it was clear this was going to be a shit storm of epic proportions. I cried, feeling I was going off to war … something I never sought. Compelled by my lifelong identity as an ICU nurse I knew I could never look back on this time with any acceptance if I succumbed to my fears for my own safety.
>
> *Nurse, intensive care, male, age 51–64*

> Fear of becoming infected with COVID will not stop me from being the best doctor I can be for the children and families I see. I didn't go to medical school to now hide from my patients in the time of a pandemic.
>
> *Senior doctor, paediatrics, female, age 41–50*

Some healthcare workers talked about feelings of pride and gratitude in having the opportunity to serve their community and using their skills to help others.

> I'm glad I'm in a job where I hopefully help people feel a little better.
>
> *Nurse, emergency department, male, age 20–30*

> I feel like my chosen career has given me the opportunity to shine at work and inspire my team.
>
> *Senior doctor, emergency department, female, age 41–50*

It has been good to be able to maintain employment during this time and to feel useful at the frontline.

Administrative worker, emergency department, female, age 51–64

I feel grateful for being able to do the work that I do.

Clinical scientist, respiratory medicine, female, age 31–40

We are lucky to come to work. To be able to do something with a group of people you like and respect that helps our patients and their families is a privilege.

Nurse, medical specialty, female, age 51–64

Mostly I feel very proud of being a nurse during this pandemic and know how useful and valuable I am to the community and know that I play a pivotal role in the fight against this pandemic.

Nurse, intensive care, female, age 41–50

I feel proud that I am a front-line worker during this pandemic, making a difference and being part of history. This is my role and I undertake it professionally.

Nurse, COVID-screening ward, female, age 51–64

I felt worried about the risk, but felt the patients who were in isolation found the situation really hard. I was happy to do what I could for them in a very difficult situation and would do it again.

Allied health practitioner, rehabilitation, female, age 51–64

Having the opportunity to work in the COVID screening clinic during the testing surge was really important to me. It made me feel useful and valuable and that I was able to actually do something to help against the pandemic, rather than just providing the reduced clinical service that we are providing in my other work, as we are only working remotely at present.

Physiotherapist, community care, female, age 31–40

It's obviously very challenging, but I feel rewarded in the sense that I'm making a positive contribution to society. I'm making use of the skills and knowledge that I have built up during my training.

Senior doctor, anaesthetics, male, age 41–50

I have learnt about adapting to unforeseen changes, about people, and about myself.

General practitioner, female, age 41–50

It's been an exciting time working in infection prevention and control. I have never felt more valued or appreciated.

Nurse, infectious diseases, female, age 51–64

> I decided to face my anxiety, and volunteer to help out a sub-acute area of nursing hit hard by COVID-19, regaining strength and confidence afterwards when I finished and remained well and COVID free. Overall, I was energised by being able to help in a time of crisis.
>
> *Nurse, surgical, female, age 31–40*

> Being on the frontline and listening to patients as they share their fears, pain, and isolation because no family visitors are allowed has been an honour and privilege.
>
> *Spiritual care, surgical, female, age 51–64*

At times, being at work was easier than being isolated at home watching the news regarding the effects of the pandemic overseas. Work offered routine, distraction, and social connection.

> The days when I was at home, especially earlier on when you were bombarded by the media were more anxiety-provoking. It was actually nice to be at work. Our ICU doctors very early provided us with a role (proning patients). I feel this gave us the feeling that we were helping somehow, which allowed me to feel I was more in control.
>
> *Physiotherapist, intensive care, female, age 20–30*

> Sometimes it actually felt more calming being at work and caring for COVID patients rather than sitting at home and watching the pandemic unfolding on the news.
>
> *Nurse, intensive care, female, age 20–30*

> Being able to go to work and spend all day with people has been the best thing for my mental health. As draining as work can be, it's incredibly fulfilling and the socialisation has prevented any serious deterioration in my mental health.
>
> *Nurse, intensive care, female, age 20–30*

> My work has been a huge saving grace for me over the past year. It is the one thing that has provided a sense of stability, order, and routine in my life. I work with a wonderful team of people who are as compassionate and supportive as they are professional. My work is highly rewarding, and I feel our work makes a huge difference to our patients/clients and their families. I am glad of my job in so many ways and thankful even when other aspects of my life seem somewhat out of control. It feels like it's the glue that's keeping things together for me.
>
> *Occupational therapist, palliative care, female, age 51–64*

> I felt most anxious before starting to work with COVID-positive patients. However, once I got into it, I have felt in control and really happy to be making a difference.
>
> *Nurse, medical specialty, female, age 41–50*

> I get to leave the house every day, come and hang out with my friends at work, work hard, feel useful, and go home again.
>
> *Senior doctor, emergency department, female, age 41–50*

> I've been inspired by the support in my workplace and the people in it. I feel it's really brought people together and let workers demonstrate skills—work and personal—in a way they maybe wouldn't have to the same degree pre COVID.
>
> *Physiotherapist, emergency department, female, age 41–50*

There was a sense of being a part of history-in-the-making.

> It has been a once in a lifetime experience I hope that what we have learnt and shared will help future healthcare workers.
>
> *Nurse, outpatients, male, age 51–64*

> Down the line, we could say to our grandchildren that: "I was a part of history, looking after patients that have been affected by this virus". Epic.
>
> *Nurse, hospital aged care, female, age 41–50*

Growth

Many healthcare workers described feelings of growth and achievement during the pandemic. They reflected on how much they had learnt about themselves, and about others, and valued the opportunity to develop new skills.

> I think encouraging staff to step forward and see this period as a time of growth can help. And celebrate the wins together—the patients that are getting better and surviving.
>
> *Nurse, intensive care, female, age 41–50*

> Having purpose and satisfaction in my work, and pursuing growth and development, has been helpful.
>
> *Psychologist, medical specialty, female, age 51–64*

> A growth mindset helped: we have seen this before and survived, let's sort out the best way through.
>
> *Senior doctor, emergency department, female, age 41–50*

> I appreciate the post-traumatic growth and shift in perspective.
>
> *Respiratory scientist, female, age 31–40*

> It's been a very good experience for me working in this pandemic. I felt it gave me more experience in dealing with hard situations and made me

stronger. It's a great feeling to be part of a team that was courageous enough to face this pandemic and accept this challenge to look after sick people, to be there until the recovery.

Nurse, hospital aged care, female, age 41–50

Gratitude

Amidst all the loss and uncertainty, healthcare workers found much to be grateful for.

Counting my blessings—stable work, a house, a family, good health, savings—has been helpful in re-setting my mindset when I start to feel overwhelmed.

Social worker, aged care psychiatry, female, age 51–64

I am one of the lucky ones who has a loving partner and family, so I am grateful for that.

Junior doctor, emergency department, female, age 31–40

The positive aspect is I am working less hours, and spending quality time at home with my family instead. So COVID is a nightmare, but I actually am thankful of where I am.

Senior doctor, anaesthetics, male, age 31–40

Teachers deserve incredible gratitude, especially newer teachers. Teaching would be such an intense job currently. A big thank you to all those involved in agriculture, transport, cleaning, cooking, trades, and all the other usually unseen occupations that our society relies on. Stay well and safe everyone!

Nurse, hospital aged care, female, age 31–40

I'm thankful that my son can continue to go to school.

Psychologist, community care, female, age 31–40

We need to remember what is truly important. Relationships, connections, experiences are what is important. Even though we may be limited in terms of movement and travel, we can still enjoy these things in different ways. Short term joys like going to a pub, going out to a restaurant, going shopping, these are all trivial, meaningless things in the long term. We are so lucky in Australia, with our climate, landscape, freedom of speech. It is all about relativity … instead of thinking about what we have lost, think about what we still have.

Junior doctor, surgical, male, age 31–40

Having a mindset of gratitude, a love of life, and acceptance that suffering is inevitable, helps all challenges.

Nurse, intensive care, female, age 51–64

I have always felt gratitude for being employed during this time and having a roof over my head and that all the people who are in my heart are safe and well.

Physiotherapist, community care, female, age 41–50

Food supplied at work has been a massive blessing. One thing not to worry about when you're trying to minimise supermarket runs and the stress of managing domestic chores.

Nurse, intensive care, female, age 31–40

Being provided with complimentary meals at work was excellent. It took a lot of stress away when working extra shifts—I didn't have to worry about groceries or cooking. Initiatives like this are really helpful and appreciated!

Nurse, intensive care, female, age 31–40

Every shift that I work I thank the Lord for living in Australia and having the wonderful health system that we have. It may have a few warts but, overall, it's pretty good. It has been good to feel supported overall by the community, with the local council making parking areas free for health care workers, free coffees, notes of appreciation from local schools.

Administrative worker, emergency department, female, age 51–64

I am thankful that I live in a walkable suburb with a park, and groceries in a walkable distance. I'm also thankful for technology to call friends and socialise online. My workplace has been so supportive and my boss puts in so much work to secure PPE and emails prompt updates, and provided good staffing ratios. For all of the above I am thankful.

Nurse, surgical, female, age 31–40

I've made some poor choices trying to comfort myself—I adopted two cats when I should have adopted just one—but, overall, my experiences have been relatively unfussed. I count my blessings.

Administrative worker, perioperative care, female, age 31–40

And for some healthcare workers, there were important life lessons gained.

There have been some positives about the experiences, I think that we may have realised a bit more about what really matters.

Administrative worker, community care, female, age 65–70

This pandemic has been a unique teacher. It has taught us many things and more importantly somewhat compelled us to reflect upon our lives. It has forcefully taught us the forgotten art of how to compromise and live with less.

Senior doctor, medical specialty, male, age 31–40

> It has made me a better person. I appreciate family and the small things now. I love life more.
>
> *Administrative worker, facilities and maintenance, female, age 41–50*

> I have learnt about adapting to unforeseen changes, about people, and about myself.
>
> *General practitioner, female, age 41–50*

Community kindness and appreciation

Healthcare workers were deeply touched by the words of encouragement, gratitude, and kindness from members of the community.

> The emails from school kids—with their art saying "thank you"—put a smile on my face.
>
> *Junior doctor, emergency department, female, age 31–40*

> Loved being thanked for our roles and it's been wonderful that many places have donated gifts and food to my COVID [screening] clinic.
>
> *Nurse, infectious diseases, female, age 41–50*

> One of the things I found most helpful was the "adopt a healthcare worker" Facebook page. It offered practical support, and well wishes from the community. A community offering practical support for healthcare workers is a wonderful idea.
>
> *General practitioner, female, age 41–50*

> Community support for nurses has helped me feel more loved and supported, and made my sacrifice to not see my family a bit easier to handle.
>
> *Nurse, hospital aged care, female, age 41–50*

A few healthcare workers expressed apprehension about community support fading as the pandemic wore on.

> At the start of the pandemic, I felt the community support was very encouraging (e.g., free coffees, discounts etc). However, I feel that with the second wave, there was not really any proper encouragement or support offered from anywhere, like the novelty of our hard work had worn off.
>
> *Nurse, medical specialty, female, age 20–30*

> As the pandemic progressed, the community also got carer's burn out, I think.
>
> *General practitioner, female, age 41–50*

Others spoke about feeling lifted up and restored by acts of kindness, such as free meals and other treats, offered by their communities during these dark and uncertain times.

> Positive feedback that we are doing a great job is great for morale. Food goods were a lovely support.
>
> *Nurse, emergency department, female, age 20–30*

> The acts of kindness from strangers. In the COVID [screening] clinic we receive such things as hand cream, meals, ice-cream from companies. It's the thought of support.
>
> *Nurse, medical specialty, female, age 51–64*

> Little things, like companies reaching out to us with care packages, really provides us with an uplifting spirit that encourages us to return to work time after time.
>
> *Nurse, medical, surgical and sub-acute, female, age 31–40*

> Treats donated to my workplace have been a highlight.
>
> *Nurse, perioperative care, female, age 51–64*

> As time has gone on, I feel the community has adapted amazingly well to supporting healthcare workers. In the area I live there have been flexible shopping arrangements for healthcare workers, many businesses and locals offering free meals to healthcare workers, and services advertised by the local council for mental health support.
>
> *Nurse, research unit, female, age 31–40*

> Some places (camping parks) were offering health care workers respite accommodation which was fabulous. To get away from city, television, and media was very refreshing.
>
> *Nurse, intensive care, female, age 51–64*

> Donations of food and goodies, and notes of encouragement from the community and local businesses, really boosted morale at work.
>
> *Nurse, intensive care, female, age 20–30*

> It feels good to know finally that the community appreciates our role and our importance, and values our job. I hope it lasts long after the pandemic.
>
> *Nurse, intensive care, female, age 41–50*

16
LOOKING BACK, LOOKING FORWARDS

> We were not prepared. The experts were warning us for decades that a pandemic was coming but we didn't listen. We have to listen to the experts better and the government shouldn't be afraid to do that either.
>
> *Nurse, infectious diseases, female, age 31–40*

Crises like the pandemic can both reveal and transform how we see our place in the world, as individuals and as communities. In this final chapter, we share healthcare workers' reflections on the pandemic, the lessons that can be learnt from this experience, and how the current pandemic can help us to prepare for future crises. Some healthcare workers drew parallels between the current crisis and past pandemics—to suggest that a stronger appreciation and understanding of history could have prepared our healthcare systems, and societies, to better respond to COVID-19. Others looked to the future, drawing connections between the pandemic and other pressing challenges facing humanity—loss of biodiversity, unsustainable growth, and failure to invest in prevention in the endless pursuit of a cure. They called for greater attention to the social and environmental determinants of health and illness. And they urged us to learn from the pandemic, to strengthen our response to other urgent global threats including climate change and widening health and social inequities.

How did we find ourselves in this position?

Healthcare workers wrote that COVID-19 was not the first global public health crisis, and would not be the last, drawing parallels with other viruses that spread globally, from the Spanish influenza virus to more recent examples including Severe Acute Respiratory Syndrome (SARS) in the early 2000s. They believed that a better

DOI: 10.4324/9781003228394-16

understanding of past pandemics would have prepared societies and healthcare systems in responding to COVID-19.

> History repeats itself—how often have you heard that?
>
> *Senior doctor, general medicine, male, age 65–70*

> I believe political agendas, clinical pragmatism, and fear for self, have combined to remove almost all humanity from our response to the pandemic. The other thing I find very troubling is that we do not seem to learn from other countries or the past. So many mistakes were repeated in too many countries throughout this pandemic. And if you read up on the events of the Spanish flu, it is clear that we failed to learn the lessons of that epidemic … It's eerie to observe how the sequence of events and the measures taken/mistakes made are so similar.
>
> *Administrative worker, medical specialty, male, age 51–64*

> When you don't know what the future holds, reading history can be very informative. I encourage all junior staff to read George Soper's article from 1918 "Lessons from the Pandemic".
>
> *Senior doctor, respiratory medicine, male, age 51–64*

> Evidence regarding healthcare worker responses during a pandemic was available (e.g., from SARS) but not considered or even sought.
>
> *Senior doctor, gynaecology, female, age 51–64*

> What would have helped? Reading the SARS Commission report from Ontario, Canada, and implementing its lessons, including the precautionary principle, listening to frontline healthcare workers, improving occupational health and safety standards, and not siloing infection prevention from occupational health and safety within healthcare settings.
>
> *Junior doctor, medical specialty, male, age 31–40*

> It would have helped if governments had read the research that came out post SARS and avian flu which highlighted the issues that have been raised with this pandemic.
>
> *Paramedic, male, age 51–64*

> I am a gay doctor and have lived almost my whole life in a minority that lives with HIV. We should look at what people living with HIV/AIDS have done to reduce stigma and blame and apply to COVID. We need community education on contact tracing: gay guys do it for STIs without blinking. Silence equals death.
>
> *Senior doctor, male, age withheld*

Some healthcare workers lamented the lack of preparedness nationally, recalling the purpose-built infectious disease hospitals that were gradually closed across Australia.

> Hospitals in these modern times have not been built for a global pandemic.
>
> *Nurse, emergency department, female, age 51–64*

> Infection control was not good enough before the pandemic.
>
> *Nurse, medical specialty, female, age 51–64*

> I laugh at my little pandemic preparation box which we need for accreditation. One box of N95 masks, a box of gloves, and a bottle of hand sanitiser ... We needed a cupboard FULL of these things.
>
> *Nurse, community care, female, age 51–64*

> Perhaps there should again be a dedicated infectious diseases hospital where patients can be concentrated in, not spread around? There used to be an infectious diseases hospital. Can this be looked into as the future COVID site?
>
> *Administrative worker, surgical, female, age 51–64*

> I really feel that as a State we are not set up for infectious diseases in our public hospitals. In the past we had an infectious disease hospital, which meant all that were positive—or suspected to have an infectious disease—could go to a place that was well equipped to serve these patients, and staff who were well versed in dealing with them. As a State I think we slipped into complacency about the dangers of infectious diseases and we are now paying the price.
>
> *Nurse, community care, female, age 51–64*

Some healthcare workers expressed deep frustration that warnings about the capacity of the healthcare system to respond to a global pandemic had been ignored.

> We have been unheard for many years when we spoke up about the absence of long-term plans to address community health responses to WHO [World Health Organisation] predicted pandemics ... and that's not even going into the woeful conditions we were aware existed within the aged care sector. These negative feelings come from a sense of powerlessness and overwhelming frustration that, if our professional and empathic voices had been heeded long ago, a lot of the systemic weaknesses COVID exploited would have been plugged long before this pandemic exposed them.
>
> *Nurse, non-binary, age 41–50*

Even after the pandemic began, healthcare workers felt that authorities were often too slow to learn from mistakes made, and actions taken, in other jurisdictions and countries.

The Australian medical system needs to open its eyes and ears to other countries' strategies and not be so endemic in our, at times arrogant, strategies. We need to examine and learn what worked in countries that were overwhelmed: relying on our own experiences seems counterintuitive and simply not good enough. We do not know what the future of this pandemic will involve, and we may be one day overwhelmed which will affect present and future frontline workers.

Nurse, intensive care, male, age 51–64

Australia has unfortunately, through its complacency, allowed a disaster in Melbourne. We need fewer talking points from politicians and bureaucrats trying to defend their legacy and more concrete actions to improve PPE, testing, tracing, isolation, staffing.

General practitioner, non-binary, age 31–40

We were playing catch-up in the way that we had to deal with new challenges both at work and in the community. There was a sense of dread with what we were seeing in the media in countries such as Spain, England and America in the initial wave. When cases started to appear in Australia there seemed to be this "wait and see" attitude from governments before imposing restrictions. COVID-19 has turned 2020 upside down in so many ways and hopefully we all learn from this.

Allied health assistant, rehabilitation, male, age 51–64

I wish the states would learn from each other—Victoria may have stuffed up hotel quarantine but New South Wales is making similar mistakes. New South Wales is doing a great job with tracing and who knows how Victoria has improved.

Senior doctor, medical specialty, female, age 31–40

It's not just what PPE is supplied, it's how it is used, and other behavioural measures. All we had to do was look to other countries who have already figured this out before, such as all facing the same direction when eating (tearooms), no talking when eating, stop thinking we need to touch to greet. We need to stop being complacent. We are still not prepared.

Senior doctor, medical specialty, female, age 31–40

I think we were lucky. There was some really good management, and some really stupid management. Allowing people out of quarantine, to roam the hospital, to visit on compassionate grounds. Poorly managed. They went to the shops. Went and grabbed a cup of coffee. Went outside for a cigarette. We were lucky.

Nurse, intensive care, female, age 51–64

Some observed that we would need to live with COVID-19 for some time, and that this would not be the last pandemic we faced.

> Continuing to deal with the restrictions, continual suspected-COVID and COVID patients, and the ever-changing policies and procedures in Melbourne has been exceptionally difficult. And it most likely won't be over for some time, which is the trickiest part to deal with. This is the new way of life for some time.
>
> *Nurse, surgical, female, age 31–40*

> Look after the hospitals and ensure they are up-to-date and built for crises because you never know when it will happen again.
>
> *Nurse, casual pool, female, age 20–30*

> We need to learn from this pandemic's mistakes and create a plan for future pandemics.
>
> *General practitioner, female, age 31–40*

Preparing for future crises

The pandemic was viewed as a critical moment for positive social change. A time to take stock and identify what changes need to be made within the healthcare system and workforce, and whether new approaches could be beneficial. A crucial lesson was the importance of adaptability, flexibility, and innovation.

> We need to stand back and assess how the changed plan or approach is working and be prepared to revise it, should it seem sub-optimal, or if you hear about another approach that might be better. As long as the team is informed and able to have input, that is likely to go better than staying with something that isn't working well.
>
> *Senior doctor, respiratory medicine, female, age 51–64*

> There should be no expectation of a perfect processes in a pandemic. Every workplace has a lot of self-reflection to do.
>
> *Nurse, general medicine, female, age 41–50*

> We need to allow the time and effort to reflect, evaluate, and hold onto the learning. So that in the event of another crisis we can transfer our learning.
>
> *Social worker, medical specialty, female, age 51–64*

> Innovative models of infection prevention should be championed instead of discredited. For example, the current guidelines are outdated and NOT

> inclusive of aerosol science, but based on tuberculosis studies which may not even stand up to the rigor of modern-day evidence evaluation.
>
> *Nurse, respiratory medicine, female, age 51–64*

> I think there are a lot of things that we will need to reflect on from this pandemic once we get a chance to catch our breath!
>
> *Senior doctor, hospital aged care, female, age 31–40*

> Having the whole medical system stretched to snapping point prior to the onset of the pandemic was asking for disaster. We need some space in the system for flexibility and flux, creating an opportunity for resilience when future crises occur.
>
> *Senior doctor, general medicine, female, age 41–50*

Healthcare workers wrote positively about the raised profile of infection control, public health, and patient safety.

> The positive thing about this all is that as a respiratory nurse there has been a burgeoning revival of how to assess, treat and analyse respiratory disease spread. We have made major improvements in culture change around nebulisation and infection spread prevention; we have been working on this for over 20 years!
>
> *Nurse, respiratory medicine, female, age 51–64*

> The pandemic has done wonders for raising the profile of epidemiology and population health.
>
> *Senior doctor, respiratory medicine, male, age 51–64*

Better preparation for crisis events included investment in public health, better planning, greater involvement of clinicians in decision-making, and more simulation-based training.

> We need increased resourcing of public health in normal times, as well as in crisis.
>
> *Senior doctor, infectious diseases, female, age 31–40*

> We need proper preparation and use of precautionary principles, not leaving it to luck and assuming we will be fine.
>
> *Senior doctor, medical specialty, female, age 31–40*

> In anticipation of likely future crisis events and pandemics we need a centralised disaster unit that incorporates primary care and hospital care across federal and state jurisdictions.
>
> *General practitioner, female, age 51–64*

We need clear strategies and battle plans from the executive and the Department of Health—proactive rather than reactive. We need to see leaders at the coal face.

Senior doctor, surgical, female, age 51–64

We need more disaster training. Or simulation programs. That way, we are regularly reminded that these things may happen and we would have an idea or basic knowledge on what to do.

Nurse, hospital aged care, female, age 31–40

We should do more simulations of high-risk procedures on COVID patients such as intubation and MET [Medical Emergency Team] calls.

Senior doctor, medical specialty, female, age 41–50

Scenario-based training to demonstrate behaviours that are supportive, and those that are not supportive or effective in crisis, may help.

Clinical scientist, general medicine, female, age 41–50

The most useful strategy we found was simulation—to develop and test processes and tools (such as cognitive aids to help with donning and doffing PPE), and to provide training. Definitely would retain and expand on both strategies for future.

Senior doctor, anaesthetics, female, age 41–50

Policies, action plans (pandemic planning), risk assessments, equipment essentials, and communication methods need to be reviewed and updated using real data to ensure we are better able to handle a situation like this in the future.

Administrative, respiratory medicine, female, age 51–64

I hope we learn from this and have things in place for the future.

Allied health practitioner, hospital aged care, female, age 51–64

On the upside, we are now more ready and prepared to be agile in future crises or events.

Clinical scientist, general medicine, female, age 41–50

A better healthcare system for health workers

Healthcare workers also wrote about the need to build a stronger and more resilient healthcare system, equipped with the resources to tackle the ongoing pandemic as well as future crises.

More funds in the system for more nurses to allow for more holistic care—instead of rushed care.

Nurse, intensive care, female, age 31–40

> We need pre-planning for peaks and strain on resources. Organisations need to be agile, and have the ability to share workforce, patient load, and resources.
>
> *Nurse, medical specialty, female, age 51–64*

> There is a fear that we won't have learnt the lessons of COVID and we'll fall back into our old ways.
>
> *Pharmacist, female, age 31–40*

Healthcare workers also called for a focus on fairness in the healthcare system to address disparities that exist across different roles, sectors, and cohorts of patients.

> Everyone deserves to be treated with fairness. Hospital frontline workers should receive some special leave when they experience such high stress, or a risk allowance for their dedication to work and community. Aged care sector and hospital sector workers should be treated equally.
>
> *Nurse, general medicine, female, age 20–30*

> Nurses have a huge amount of responsibility within the healthcare system while having relatively low levels of respect and remuneration. This has certainly been highlighted in the pandemic and continues to be an ongoing issue. More respect from colleagues and the community can only be gained by increasing the professional status of nurses through education and improved financial remuneration.
>
> *Nurse, research institute, female, age 20–30*

> It is a disgrace that, even in normal times, nurses had to strike or campaign to get $1 or $2 pay increments.
>
> *Nurse, medical specialty, male, age 31–40*

> I suspect that if nurses were predominantly male, the pay rates would be higher.
>
> *Psychologist, hospital aged care, female, age 51–64*

> What would help? Additional paid leave. Flexibility with working hours. Recognition of allied health staff, not just doctors and nurses.
>
> *Occupational therapist, medical specialty, female, age 20–30*

> We need better gender equity measures to support female leadership.
>
> *Senior doctor, emergency medicine, female, age 41–50*

Across the health sector, the pandemic shone a spotlight on workplace safety. Some healthcare workers expressed a hope that this focus on safe workplaces would be sustained beyond the end of the pandemic.

> I am optimistic that this pandemic will highlight the role of the occupational health and safety units, and that they will be given a genuine voice at the table of pretty much every decision in hospitals.
>
> *Speech pathologist, medical specialty, female, age 41–50*

> Healthcare organisations need to do more (and earlier) to ensure extra staffing and training so that staff feel protected and safe when going to work.
>
> *Nurse, emergency department, female, age 20–30*

A more equitable and just society

Healthcare workers also wrote about how the pandemic starkly exposed health, social, and economic inequalities that have long-existed in Australian society.

> A myriad of socioeconomic inequities has been exposed during this time of global crisis.
>
> *Nurse, community care, female, age 31–40*

> Social injustice is hard to watch.
>
> *Senior doctor, surgical, male, age 41–50*

> I worried about how people who were less fortunate than me were coping. Those who lost their employment. I worry about the growing inequity in Australia.
>
> *Nurse, community care, female, age 51–64*

> A lot of stress is generated from seeing the gaps in our safety net health care system glaringly. And how slowly and imperfectly it felt things were implemented for our most vulnerable communities.
>
> *Junior doctor, general medicine, female, age 31–40*

> I hope that our elderly in aged or residential care never again have to experience such isolation and vulnerability; that we are better able to protect them and provide them with the care they deserve.
>
> *Nurse, surgical, female, age 51–64*

> We need a government who realises our society is only as well as our most vulnerable population (the elderly, the disabled, the mentally unwell), and so works to better resource services.
>
> *Nurse, emergency department, female, age 31–40*

National and global health challenges

For many healthcare workers, the pandemic called to mind the broader global challenges of the 21st century, and raised deep concerns about the aptitude of national and international leaders to respond to these issues.

> This pandemic has increased my distress about broader societal issues.
>
> *Occupational therapist, community care, female, age 51–64*

> Global warming is our biggest public health challenge. We need the government and its health departments to acknowledge the connection between global warming and the present crisis.
>
> *Nurse, surgical, male, age 51–64*

> My main source of anxiety and depression is the climate crisis. Yet, COVID has tragically side-lined this bigger issue for now, while also making me increasingly despair regarding humanity's response to existential threats.
>
> *Senior doctor, palliative care, female, age 41–50*

> The narrative of the cause of the pandemic should include deforestation which is also contributing to global warming.
>
> *Nurse, surgical, male, age 51–64*

Some healthcare workers expressed a sense of hopelessness about the situation, and what the pandemic indicated about our capacity (or lack thereof) as a global society to act collectively in times of crisis.

> I have a lower threshold for feeling angry about other important issues—most particularly climate change, refugees, treatment of animals. I despair for humanity more often than I used to, and feel less optimistic that the world can adapt to change when there is no cohesion globally—geopolitically much feels hopeless and COVID has amplified this.
>
> *Nurse, palliative care, female, age 51–64*

> Let's get away from the bullshit "frontline healthcare workers are heroes" narrative, and use the pandemic as an opportunity to focus on the real issues concerning public health: deforestation, global warming, a rapacious free market ideology that drives inequity and poor health outcomes.
>
> *Nurse, surgical, male, age 51–64*

> I feel like my hope for the future has been reduced.
>
> *Social worker, emergency department, female, age 41–50*

> We have had three novel coronaviruses since 2003. It feels inevitable that we will have another within the next decade. I feel like governments are more concerned about getting re-elected. I am just glad I have money and my family, the rest feels inevitable.
>
> *Senior doctor, hospital aged care, female, age 41–50*

> I'm more concerned about broader societal issues—dominance of self-interest and what the pandemic has exposed regarding capacity of governments to

cope with major challenges like climate change. It makes me fearful for the health of people and the environment.

Occupational therapist, community care, female, age 51–64

I have given up on any of the problems this pandemic has exposed or created ever being fixed.

Junior doctor, intensive care, male, age 31–40

I have difficulty thinking about the climate that my grandchildren will grow up in. Will this become the new "norm" and what implications for society as a whole will that have?

Allied health practitioner, medical specialty, female, age 65–70

Finally, healthcare workers wrote about the need to move towards a fairer, more ethical, and more cohesive society.

Social health and a more cohesive society and respectful government, e.g. the kind, calm, respectful and responsible, and socially and environmentally responsible of New Zealand, would be great!

Psychologist, palliative care, female, age 51–64

Social care is an important part of the health system: housing, parenting, education, employment, health literacy, system literacy, community connectedness. Social care has an important part to play and we need to tap into this.

General practitioner, male, age 51–64

We need solidarity behind public health messages and push back against partisan politicisation of health.

General practitioner, female, age 51–64

I think education of the next generation of children is important in how they are going to deal with challenges like this in the future. We need to think about and prepare for "when" the next great psycho-social-economic challenge is going to come … not "if".

Junior doctor, emergency department, male, age 20–30

It's been challenging, we have learnt a lot, changed a lot, and in the end, I am sure there will be some positives which come out of this!

Dietician, intensive care, female, age 31–40

This experience is teaching us a lot. If we're willing to learn from it.

Nurse, hospital aged care, male, age 51–64

POSTSCRIPT

To whoever is reading this

> Don't underestimate the value of someone who simply asks, "how are you?" and listens to your answer.
>
> *Social worker, general medicine, female, age 41–50*

By the middle of 2021, over four million people around the world had died from COVID-19, including many tens of thousands of healthcare workers. Undoubtedly, many more will die. We are still too close to the event to take the full measure of it. If you are a healthcare worker, the pandemic may still feel like a complex tangle of experiences, memories, and emotions. Many of you placed your lives in the path of the disease, without the support or protection that you were owed. We hope that some of the stories shared in the book will help with making sense of your experiences, feeling less alone with your memories, and giving words to your emotions.

If you are a healthcare leader—whether that be in a formal leadership role or simply as someone who believes that things can be better and wants to be a part of that change—we hope that this book will inspire you to keep working towards a stronger, kinder, and fairer health system for our future.

And finally, if you are someone who cares about a healthcare worker—as a family member, neighbour, or friend (and isn't that perhaps all of us?)—we thank you for reading, and we hope that hearing the voices of healthcare workers will give you a deeper understanding of their pandemic experience.

> Thank you for taking the time to care about us and our well-being.
>
> *Nurse, surgical, female, age 20–30*

> Thank you for collating this feedback—it is the first time anyone has asked me.
>
> *Speech pathologist, hospital aged care, female, age 20–30*

DOI: 10.4324/9781003228394-17

Thank you for this survey. I already feel better.

Senior doctor, emergency department, male, age 51–64

My situation has not changed. However, I feel a bit better after taking this survey.

Nurse, medical specialty, female, age 51–64

Answering your questions has made me reflect on what I need to do to improve my mood and then to act on it.

Nurse, female, age 65–70

It's taken until six months into this pandemic, and perhaps until now completing this survey, to realise the impact this is having on mental health, I think as healthcare workers we push through and feel we are doing OK as we are busy.

Speech pathologist, medical specialty, female, age 31–40

This [survey] is more help than I have received from my workplace in regards my mental health in relation to COVID.

Therapist, residential aged care, female, age 41–50

Thank you for doing this research and taking health care workers into consideration.

Pharmacist, female, age 31–40

Thank you for your research. I hope these learnings are reviewed and improvement initiatives instigated.

Nurse, emergency department, female, age 41–50

I think this research is an excellent idea to quantify impacts that aren't quantifiable.

Nurse, intensive care, female, age 20–30

Thank you for surveying frontline healthcare workers. Your findings will be very interesting and hopefully reveal the extent of this pandemic's effect.

Senior doctor, hospital aged care, male, age 41–50

Thank you for doing this research to hopefully improve our systems and responses. I hope it helps.

Nurse, emergency department, female, age 20–30

I hope this survey gives you insight into how health care professionals have been dealing with this pandemic. It's been a shock to everyone and everyone is trying to navigate it.

Nurse, intensive care, female, age 20–30

All the best in the survey! I am astounded at your response numbers! Something amazing will come out of this work so—thank you!

Occupational therapist, community care, female, age 31–40

I hope you can make some positive changes for the better to support us!

Occupational therapist, hospital aged care, female, age 31–40

To whoever is reading this, please take care of yourself and people you love and care for. Your family, friends, patients. We will all get through this together.

Junior doctor, emergency department, female, age 20–30

INDEX